RING THERAPY: A GUIDE TO HEALING AND BALANCE

Dr. Constance Santego

Maximillian Enterprises
Kelowna, BC

RINGS THERAPY: A GUIDE TO HEALING AND BALANCE

Copyright © 2024 by Constance Santego.

Copy Editor & Interior Design: Constance Santego
Book Layout: ©2017 BookDesignTemplates.com
Cover Design: Jennifer Louie

Ordering Information:
Quantity sales. Special discounts are available on quantity purchases by corporations, associations, and others. For details, contact the "Special Sales Department" at the address above.

Trade Paperback ISBN: 978-1-990062-37-7
eBook ISBN 978-1-990062-38-4
Created and published In Canada. Printed and bound in the United States of America

First Edition
Published by Maximillian Enterprises
Kelowna, BC
Canada
www.constancesantego.ca

Dedication to
Joseph Ranallo, BA (Hon), MA, R. Ac.

Shift Happens…Create Magic!

—Dr.Constance Santego

ALSO BY DR. CONSTANCE SANTEGO

FICTION
The Nine Spiritual Gifts Series:
Journey of a Soul – (Vol 1 Michael)
Language of a Soul – (Vol 2 Gabriel)
Prophecy of a Soul – (Vol 3 Bath Kol)
Healing of a Soul – (Vol 4 Raphael)
Miracles of a Soul – (Vol 5 Hamied)
Knowledge of a Soul – (Vol 6 Raziel)

NONFICTION
The Intuitive Life, The Gift of Prophecy, Third Edition
Fairy Tales, Dreams and Reality… Where Are You On Your Path? Second Edition
Your Persona… The Mask You Wear
Angelic Lifestyle, A Vibrant Lifestyle
Angelic Lifestyle 42-Day Energy Cleanse
Archangel Michael's Soul Retrieval Guide
Tesla and the Future of Energy Medicine
Scaling Beyond 6 Figures: *Strategies for Health & Wellness Professionals*
Beyond the Mind: *Harnessing the Power of Astral Projection for Creative Awakening*
Bend, Don't Break: *Finding Your Way Back to Abundance*

SECRETS OF A HEALER, SERIES:
Magic Of Aromatherapy (Vol I)
Magic Of Reflexology (Vol II)
Magic Of The Gifts (Vol III)
Magic Of Muscle Testing (Vol IV)
Magic Of Iridology (Vol V)
Magic Of Massage (Vol VI)
Magic Of Hypnotherapy (Vol VII)
Magic Of Reiki (Vol VIII)
Magic Of Advanced Aromatherapy (Vol IX)
Magic Of Esthetics (Vol X)
Reiki Master's Manual (Vol XI)

ADULT COLORING JOURNALS

SERIES - ZEN COLORING:
Quantum Energy and Mindful Living Journal (Vol 1)
Reiki Energy Journal (Vol 2)
Nine Spiritual Gifts Journal (Vol 3)
I Forgive Journal (Vol 4)

SERIES – COLORING PROSPERITY:
Genie-Inspired Mandalas and Wealth Journal (Vol 1)
Entrepreneurial Mindset Reboot (Vol 2)

SERIES – HARMONIC MIND CODE:
Harmonic Mind Code Coloring Journal (Vol 1)

FOR CHILDREN
I am Big Tonight. I Don't Need the Light!

COOKBOOK
My Favorite Recipes, with a Hint of Giggle

Preface

INTRODUCTION

Welcome to a journey through the ancient wisdom of Traditional Chinese Medicine (TCM), Ayurveda, and holistic health practices. This book aims to explore the fascinating intersection of these time-honored traditions and their insights into using metals and ring placement to support and balance various conditions and body systems.

INTEGRATING TCM, AYURVEDA, AND HOLISTIC PRACTICES

Traditional Chinese Medicine (TCM): TCM is a comprehensive medical system that has been practiced for thousands of years. It emphasizes the balance of Qi (vital energy) and the harmonious interaction of the Five Elements (Wood, Fire, Earth, Metal, and Water). To restore and maintain health, TCM practitioners use various methods, including acupuncture, herbal medicine, and Qi Gong. This book will delve into how TCM principles guide using metals like gold, silver, and copper to support specific organs and energy pathways.

Ayurveda: Ayurveda, the ancient healing system from India, focuses on balancing the three doshas (Vata, Pitta, and Kapha) to achieve optimal health. This holistic approach includes diet, lifestyle, herbal remedies, and bodywork to promote physical, mental, and spiritual well-being. We will explore how Ayurveda utilizes metals such as gold, silver, and copper for their therapeutic properties and how these practices can be integrated into modern wellness routines.

Holistic Health Practices: Holistic health practices consider the whole person—body, mind, and spirit—to pursue optimal health and wellness. This approach draws from various traditions, including TCM and Ayurveda, to create a comprehensive view of health. This book will look at how holistic practices can be applied to using metal rings and finger placements to balance energy and support various body systems.

PURPOSE OF THIS BOOK

This book serves as a practical guide for those interested in exploring the benefits of metal therapy through the lens of TCM, Ayurveda, and holistic health practices. By combining these ancient traditions, we aim to comprehensively understand how metals and their strategic placement on specific fingers can influence health and well-being.

WHAT YOU WILL LEARN

- The Fundamentals: Gain a foundational understanding of TCM, Ayurveda, and holistic health principles related to metal therapy.
- Metal Properties: Discover the unique properties and health benefits of different metals such as gold, silver, copper, titanium, and nickel.
- Finger Placement: Learn the significance of wearing metal rings on specific fingers to target different body systems and conditions.
- Practical Applications: Get valuable tips and step-by-step guides for muscle testing to determine the best metal and finger placement for your individual needs.
- Scientific and Anecdotal Evidence: Explore scientific studies and traditional anecdotes supporting the use of metals in health practices.

How to Use This Book

Each chapter is designed to be informative and practical, offering insights and actionable steps that you can incorporate into your daily life. Whether you are a seasoned holistic health practitioner or new to these concepts, this book provides valuable information that can help you enhance your well-being through the strategic use of metal rings.

Join us as we bridge the wisdom of the past with the needs of the present, creating a holistic approach to health and wellness through the power of metals and mindful ring placement.

Important Notice on Liability and Consulting a Doctor

Disclaimer

The information provided in this book is intended for educational purposes only and should not be considered medical advice. The practices and suggestions described herein, including the use of metals such as silver and copper for health purposes, are based on traditional knowledge and contemporary applications. They are not intended to diagnose, treat, cure, or prevent any disease.

Liability

The author and publisher of this book assume no responsibility for any adverse effects, injuries, or damages that may result from the use or misuse of the information contained herein. Readers are strongly advised to use their own judgment and discretion when applying the practices discussed in this book.

Consulting a Doctor

Before beginning any new health regimen, incorporating supplements, or using alternative healing practices such as those described in this book, consulting with a qualified healthcare provider is crucial. This is especially important for individuals with pre-existing health conditions, those who are pregnant or breastfeeding, and those currently taking medications.

Your healthcare provider can offer personalized advice and ensure that any new practices are safe and appropriate for your specific health needs. They can also provide guidance on proper dosages and monitor for potential interactions with other treatments you may be undergoing.

Safety First

While traditional practices offer valuable insights into health and wellness, modern medical guidance is essential to ensure your safety and well-being. Always prioritize professional medical advice and support when considering changes to your health routine.

By consulting with your healthcare provider and using this book as a supplementary resource, you can make informed decisions that contribute to your overall health and well-being.

Dr. Constance Santego

Contents

Ring Therapy

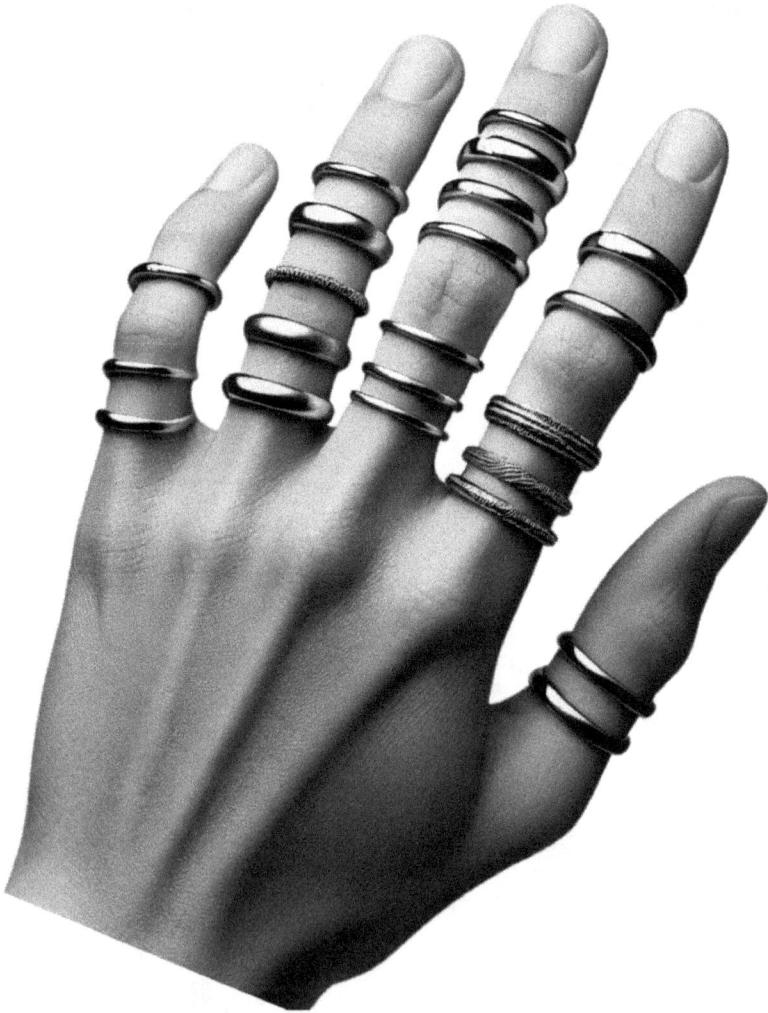

Dr. Constance Santego

Chapter 1: Introduction

Historical Perspectives on Metals in Healing

Metals have played a crucial role in the development of human civilizations, serving not only as materials for tools and currency but also as significant components in medical and spiritual practices. Here's a detailed look into how different cultures historically utilized metals for healing and their symbolic importance.

ANCIENT EGYPT

Copper: Egyptians used copper for its antibacterial properties. It was commonly used to sterilize wounds and drinking water. Copper tools and containers have been found in ancient tombs, signifying their importance in daily life and afterlife rituals.

Gold: Gold was associated with the gods and immortality. It was used in jewelry and amulets, believed to protect the wearer and bring health. The ancient Egyptians also used gold in their advanced medical practices, including dentistry.

ANCIENT GREECE AND ROME

Silver: Both Greeks and Romans recognized the antimicrobial properties of silver. They used silver containers to keep liquids fresh and prevent spoilage. Hippocrates, the "father of medicine," wrote about the healing properties of silver in wound care.

Mercury: While now known to be toxic, mercury was used by the ancient Greeks and Romans for its medicinal properties, particularly in treating skin conditions and as a component of various ointments.

ALCHEMY

Medieval Europe and the Islamic World: Alchemy, a precursor to modern chemistry, focused on the transmutation of base metals into noble metals like gold and the pursuit of the philosopher's stone, which was believed to grant immortality and heal all diseases. Alchemists in medieval Europe and the Islamic world made significant contributions to the study of metals and their properties.

NATIVE AMERICAN CULTURES

Copper: Native American tribes, particularly those around the Great Lakes, used copper for making tools, jewelry, and ceremonial objects. Copper was valued for its workability and believed spiritual properties.

Silver: Among various tribes, silver was used in jewelry and was believed to have protective and healing properties.

TRADITIONAL CHINESE MEDICINE (TCM)
Background

Origins: Emerging over 2,500 years ago, TCM is a comprehensive system of health care that encompasses a wide range of practices, including herbal medicine, acupuncture, massage, exercise, and dietary therapy. Its foundation lies in the belief that the human body is a microcosm of the universe governed by natural laws.

Philosophical Foundations: Central to TCM is the Taoist philosophy, which emphasizes living in harmony with the Tao (the Way), balancing the dualistic nature of Yin and Yang, and ensuring the smooth flow of Qi (vital energy) through the body's meridians (energy channels).

Key Concepts

Qi (Chi): Qi is the vital life force that permeates every aspect of being. The free and balanced flow of Qi is essential for health, while blockages or imbalances can lead to illness.

Yin and Yang: These are the fundamental principles of duality in TCM. Yin is characterized by qualities such as cold, rest, and passivity, whereas Yang is associated with heat, activity, and dynamism. Health is achieved by maintaining a balance between Yin and Yang.

Five Elements: Wood, Fire, Earth, Metal, and Water. These elements correspond to different organs and systems within the body and are used to diagnose and treat various health issues by understanding their interactions and balances.

Use of Metals in TCM

Gold and Silver: In TCM, gold and silver are not just precious metals but also potent therapeutic agents. Gold, associated with the Yang quality, is believed to invigorate and stimulate energy, making it ideal for tonifying and strengthening. Silver, on the other hand, with its Yin properties, is known for its calming and cooling effects, often used to clear heat and toxins from the body.

Medicinal Uses: Historically, metals such as mercury, arsenic, and lead were used in small, controlled doses within various medicinal compounds. These metals were thought to possess unique properties that could address specific imbalances, though modern TCM practices have largely moved away from these due to toxicity concerns.

AYURVEDA
Background

Origins: Ayurveda, originating in India over 3,000 years ago, is one of the world's oldest holistic healing systems. It is based on the principles found in the Vedas, ancient scriptures that provide a profound understanding of the natural world and human life.

Philosophical Foundations: Ayurveda emphasizes the interconnectedness of the body, mind, and spirit, advocating for a balanced lifestyle that harmonizes these elements with the environment. The core principle of Ayurveda is to maintain health by keeping the body's doshas (biological energies) in balance.

Key Concepts

Doshas: Vata (air and ether), Pitta (fire and water), and Kapha (water and earth). Each individual has a unique combination of these doshas, known as their prakriti. Health in Ayurveda is maintained by balancing these doshas according to one's prakriti.

Prakriti: This refers to an individual's constitution, which is determined at birth. Understanding one's prakriti helps in personalizing treatments and lifestyle choices to maintain optimal health.

Dhatus: The seven tissues that make up the body, including blood, muscle, fat, bone, marrow, semen, and plasma. Proper nourishment and balance of these tissues are crucial for health.

Use of Metals in Ayurveda

Bhasma: Ayurveda employs a unique method of preparing metals and minerals called bhasma. These are finely powdered forms of purified metals, such as Swarna Bhasma (gold), Rajata Bhasma (silver), and Parada (mercury). These preparations are believed to enhance longevity, vitality, and overall health.

Rasayana: This rejuvenation therapy often includes metallic preparations that are thought to enhance physical and mental resilience, promote longevity, and restore youthfulness.

Modern Perspectives on Metal-Based Therapies

Metal-based therapies, which have roots in ancient practices, are being revisited and explored through the lens of modern science. These therapies encompass a range of applications, from antimicrobial treatments to advanced medical procedures. Here's an overview to help you understand the contemporary approach to using metals in medicine.

Antimicrobial Properties of Metals

Silver:

Usage: Silver is renowned for its antimicrobial properties. It is used in wound dressings, coatings for medical devices, and water purification systems.

Mechanism: Silver ions disrupt bacterial cell walls, interfering with their DNA and preventing replication.

Applications: Silver sulfadiazine cream is widely used for burn wounds to prevent infections. Silver-embedded bandages and catheters reduce the risk of infections in medical settings.

Gold Nanoparticles in Medicine

Gold:

Usage: Gold nanoparticles are employed in diagnostics, drug delivery, and cancer treatment.

Mechanism: Their small size allows them to penetrate cells easily, and they can be coated with drugs or targeting molecules to deliver treatments directly to diseased cells.

Applications: Gold nanoparticles are used in imaging techniques for early detection of diseases and in photothermal therapy, where they help destroy cancer cells when exposed to specific wavelengths of light.

Titanium in Orthopedics

Titanium:

Usage: Titanium is used extensively in orthopedic implants and dental implants due to its strength, light weight, and biocompatibility.

Mechanism: Titanium is non-reactive with bodily fluids and tissues, reducing the risk of rejection and promoting bone growth around the implant.

Applications: Commonly used in hip and knee replacements, spinal fusion surgeries, and dental prosthetics.

Platinum in Chemotherapy

Platinum:

Usage: Platinum-based drugs, such as cisplatin, are widely used in chemotherapy to treat various cancers.

Mechanism: These drugs form cross-links with DNA in cancer cells, disrupting their replication and leading to cell death.

Applications: Effective in treating testicular, ovarian, lung, bladder, and other types of cancers.

Emerging Research and Future Directions

Nanotechnology:

Overview: The field of nanotechnology is expanding the use of metals in medicine, particularly through the development of metal nanoparticles for targeted therapies.

Research Focus: Current research explores metal nanoparticle use in early disease detection, personalized medicine, and regenerative medicine.

Integrative Medicine:

Overview: Integrative medicine combines conventional treatments with alternative therapies, including the use of metals.

Approach: Practitioners are looking at how traditional metal-based therapies can complement modern medical treatments to enhance efficacy and patient outcomes.

Modern perspectives on metal-based therapies demonstrate a fascinating blend of ancient wisdom and cutting-edge science. While traditional practices laid the groundwork, contemporary research continues to uncover the potential of metals in promoting health and treating diseases. As a student, understanding these developments can provide insights into how holistic and scientific approaches can converge to advance medical care.

Placebo vs. Metal Ring Therapy: Understanding the Difference

Placebo Effect: The placebo effect occurs when a person experiences a perceived improvement in their condition after receiving a treatment that has no therapeutic effect. This phenomenon is driven by the individual's belief in the treatment's efficacy, rather than any inherent properties of the treatment itself. Placebos are often used in clinical trials to test the effectiveness of new treatments, serving as a control to compare against the actual drug or therapy. While the placebo effect can lead to real improvements in symptoms, it relies entirely on psychological factors and the power of suggestion.

Metal Ring Therapy: Metal ring therapy, on the other hand, is a holistic healing practice that involves wearing metal rings on specific fingers to influence various aspects of health and well-being. This approach is based on principles from Traditional Chinese Medicine (TCM), Ayurveda, and modern holistic practices. Each metal is believed to have unique properties that can affect the body's energy flow, balance, and overall health. For instance, gold is thought to energize and support heart health, while silver is believed to have antimicrobial and calming effects. The placement of these rings on specific fingers is intended to interact with meridians and energy pathways in the body, promoting healing and balance.

Key Differences:

1. Mechanism of Action:
     - Placebo: Relies on psychological factors and the individual's belief in the treatment.
     - Metal Ring Therapy: Based on the intrinsic properties of different metals and their interaction with the body's energy systems.

2. Intent and Application:
   - o Placebo: Used primarily in clinical trials as a control to measure the effectiveness of new treatments.
   - o Metal Ring Therapy: Practiced as a complementary therapy to promote holistic health and balance, integrating traditional and modern healing principles.
3. Effectiveness:
   - o Placebo: Can lead to perceived improvements due to psychological factors, but lacks therapeutic properties.
   - o Metal Ring Therapy: Claims to offer therapeutic benefits based on the specific properties of metals and their targeted application on the body.
4. Scientific Basis:
   - o Placebo: Well-documented and widely studied in the context of clinical research.
   - o Metal Ring Therapy: Rooted in traditional practices and holistic theories, with varying levels of scientific validation.

While the placebo effect demonstrates the power of the mind in healing, metal ring therapy aims to harness the unique properties of metals to provide tangible health benefits. Both approaches highlight the complex interplay between belief, perception, and physical health.

Chapter 2: Metals

Absorption of Metals Through the Skin and Its Impact on Health

The idea that wearing metal rings can affect your health is based on the skin's ability to absorb small amounts of metals. Here's a simplified explanation:

How Metals Are Absorbed

> Skin Permeability: The skin can absorb small amounts of substances, including metals. Factors like sweat, skin condition, and how long you wear the ring can affect absorption.
>
> Interaction with Sweat and Oil: Sweat and natural oils (sebum) on your skin can help transfer metal ions from the ring into your body.
>
> Micro-abrasions and Contact: Small cuts or prolonged contact with metal can enhance absorption.

Potential Risks

> Metal Sensitivity: Some people might have allergic reactions, like redness or itching.

Toxicity: Excessive exposure to metals can be harmful, so it's important to use high-quality metals and not overdo it.

Practical Tips

Monitor Your Skin: Watch for any signs of irritation or allergic reactions.

Use Quality Metals: Ensure you are using pure, non-reactive metals.

Re-evaluate Regularly: Check how your body responds and adjust as needed.

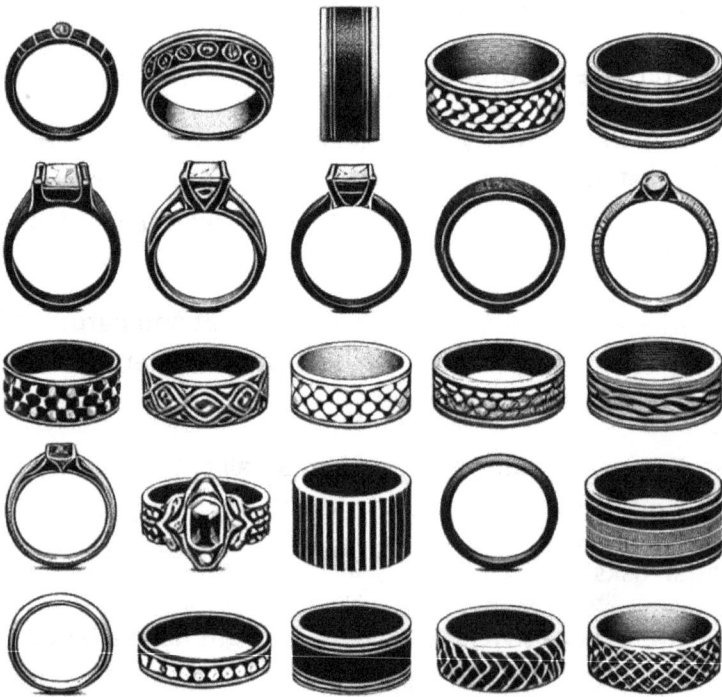

The Potential Negativity of Wearing Metal Rings with Diamonds or Gemstones

While metal rings have been used for centuries for their healing properties, the inclusion of diamonds or other gemstones in the rings can introduce certain negative influences. Understanding these potential issues is important for those seeking to use metal rings for holistic healing.

Diamonds

Emotional Baggage: Diamonds are believed to retain and hold onto emotional energies and experiences from all previous wearers. This can include both positive and negative emotions, which may affect the current wearer.

Inability to Clear: Unlike some other crystals and gemstones, diamonds are considered difficult to cleanse of their accumulated emotional energies. This persistent energy can influence or override the intended benefits of the metal ring.

Intensification of Energies: Diamonds are known to amplify energies. If not properly cleansed, they may intensify negative emotions or unresolved issues from past wearers, impacting the current wearer's emotional balance and well-being.

Other Gemstones

Emotional Constituents: Each gemstone has its unique emotional properties, which can affect the wearer differently. For example:

- Amethyst: Known for its calming properties but may hold onto the anxiety and stress aggression from past use, previous users, and if not properly cleansed.
- Emerald: Associated with love and compassion but may retain emotional pain aggression from past use, previous users, and if not properly cleansed.
- Ruby: Symbolizes passion and vitality but can also amplify anger or aggression from past use and previous users if not properly cleansed.
- Sapphire: Represents wisdom and clarity yet may carry confusion, sadness, and aggression from past use and previous users if not properly cleansed.
- Energy Residue: Like diamonds, many gemstones can hold onto the energies of those who wore them before. This residual energy can influence the new wearer, potentially causing emotional imbalances or other negative effects.

Cleaning Difficulties: While some gemstones can be cleansed more easily than diamonds, they still require regular and thorough cleaning to remove any residual emotional energies. Failure to do so can result in the stone influencing the wearer in unintended ways.

Metals and Their Uses in TCM, Ayurveda, and Holistic Practices

GOLD

PROPERTIES AND BENEFITS OF GOLD
Chemical Stability:

> Durability: Gold is highly resistant to corrosion and oxidation. This stability makes it an excellent material for long-term use in medical devices and implants.

Conductivity:

> Electrical and Thermal Conductivity: Gold is an excellent conductor of electricity and heat. This property is useful in electronics and medical devices where reliable electrical connections are necessary.

Biocompatibility:

> Non-reactive Nature: Gold is biocompatible, meaning it does not cause adverse reactions when used in the body. This property is crucial for medical implants and devices that need to interact with body tissues without causing inflammation or rejection.

Anti-inflammatory Properties:

> Therapeutic Use: Gold compounds have anti-inflammatory properties, which are beneficial in treating conditions like rheumatoid arthritis. This property helps reduce inflammation, which can also indirectly benefit the circulatory system by reducing inflammation-related damage to blood vessels.

Traditional Chinese Medicine (TCM):

- Properties: Warm and tonifying.
- Uses: Used in acupuncture needles and certain herbal formulations to strengthen the body's yang energy, improve circulation, and enhance mental clarity.
- Balancing Elements: Often used to tonify and strengthen the Fire element (Heart), which supports vitality and energy.

Ayurveda:

- Properties: Rejuvenating and strengthening.
- Uses: Used in rasayana (rejuvenation) therapies to enhance vitality, immunity, and longevity.
    - Balancing Elements: Primarily balances Pitta (Fire) and Vata (Air and Ether) by promoting warmth and energy.

Holistic Practices:

- Benefits: Enhances emotional stability, supports heart health, and promotes overall vitality.
- Finger Placement: Commonly worn on the ring finger to influence the heart and emotional balance.

SILVER

PROPERTIES AND BENEFITS OF SILVER

Silver is a precious metal with a long history of use in medicine and healing. It is known for its antimicrobial properties, making it effective against a wide range of bacteria, viruses, and fungi. Let's delve into the properties and benefits of silver, especially in relation to the respiratory system.

Properties of Silver

> Antimicrobial: Silver has powerful antimicrobial properties. It can kill or inhibit the growth of bacteria, viruses, and fungi. This makes it valuable in preventing and treating infections.

> Anti-Inflammatory: Silver has anti-inflammatory effects, which can help reduce swelling and irritation in the respiratory tract.

> Healing: Silver promotes the healing of tissues. It has been used in wound dressings and medical devices to aid in recovery and prevent infections.

> Conductivity: Silver is an excellent conductor of electricity and heat. While this property is more relevant in technology, it underscores the metal's unique nature.

Traditional Chinese Medicine (TCM):

- Properties: Cooling and calming.
- Uses: Commonly used in acupuncture needles and topical applications for its antimicrobial properties.

- Balancing Elements: Used to disperse excess heat, calming the Fire element and supporting the Metal element (Lungs) by clearing heat and toxins.

Ayurveda:

- Properties: Cooling and calming.
- Uses: Used in formulations for mental clarity, emotional stability, and to treat conditions like anxiety and insomnia.
- Balancing Elements: Balances Pitta (Fire) by providing a cooling effect, also calming Vata.

Holistic Practices:

- Benefits: Supports respiratory health, reduces infections, and promotes mental clarity.
- Finger Placement: Often worn on the little finger for respiratory benefits and on the ring finger for skin health.

COPPER

PROPERTIES AND BENEFITS OF COPPER

Copper is a versatile and essential metal with a rich history of use in various cultures for its healing properties. Known for its excellent conductivity and anti-inflammatory effects, copper plays a crucial role in supporting the circulatory system. Its unique properties make it beneficial in medical applications, dietary supplements, and wearable health accessories. Let's explore the properties and benefits of copper, especially in relation to the heart and blood vessels.

Properties of Copper

Anti-inflammatory Properties: Therapeutic Use: Copper has well-known anti-inflammatory properties. It is often used to reduce inflammation in conditions such as arthritis. By reducing inflammation, copper can help alleviate stress on the blood vessels, thereby supporting overall circulatory health.

Antioxidant Activity: Free Radical Neutralization: Copper acts as an antioxidant, neutralizing free radicals that can damage cells and tissues. This property is crucial for protecting the heart and blood vessels from oxidative stress, which can lead to cardiovascular diseases.

Essential Nutrient: Role in Hemoglobin Formation: Copper is essential for the formation of hemoglobin, the protein in red blood cells that carries oxygen throughout the body. Adequate copper levels ensure efficient oxygen transport, which is vital for maintaining healthy circulation.

Iron Absorption: Copper aids in the absorption of iron, another essential mineral for blood health. This synergistic effect ensures that the body maintains a balanced level of vital nutrients necessary for a robust circulatory system.

Anti-microbial Properties: Hygiene and Health: Copper has natural antimicrobial properties that help prevent infections. This property is particularly beneficial in medical settings where copper is used in surfaces and devices to reduce the risk of bacterial and viral contamination.

Conductivity: Electrical and Thermal Conductivity: Copper is a superb conductor of electricity and heat. This property makes it useful in various medical devices and applications where efficient electrical conduction is required.

Blood Flow Support: The excellent conductivity of copper helps enhance the flow of energy through the body, supporting the circulatory system.

Traditional Chinese Medicine (TCM):

- Properties: Warming and conductive.
- Uses: Used in TCM tools and sometimes in topical formulations.
- Balancing Elements: Supports the Liver (Wood) and promotes the smooth flow of Qi, addressing stagnation.

Ayurveda:

- Properties: Warming and stimulating.
- Uses: Used to enhance digestion and metabolism, treat liver disorders, and support the cardiovascular system.

- Balancing Elements: Balances Kapha (Earth and Water) by promoting heat and movement, also supporting Pitta.

Holistic Practices:

- Benefits: Reduces inflammation, supports digestive health, and enhances joint health.
- Finger Placement: Commonly worn on the ring finger for digestive and circulatory benefits.

STAINLESS STEEL

PROPERTIES AND BENEFITS OF STAINLESS STEEL

Stainless steel is a modern marvel in the realm of metals, known for its exceptional durability, resistance to corrosion, and hypoallergenic properties. It has become a staple in various medical applications and wearable health accessories due to its safety and longevity. Its non-reactive nature makes it suitable for individuals with metal sensitivities. Let's delve into the properties and benefits of stainless steel, particularly in its role supporting general health and medical applications.

Properties of Stainless Steel

Chemical Properties:

Durability and Strength: High Strength: Stainless steel is renowned for its high strength and durability, making it an excellent choice for medical devices and implants that require long-term use.

Corrosion Resistance: The addition of chromium to stainless steel enhances its resistance to corrosion, ensuring longevity even in harsh environments, such as inside the human body.

Biocompatibility: Non-reactive Surface: Stainless steel is biocompatible, meaning it does not cause adverse reactions when in contact with biological tissues. This property is crucial for medical implants and devices that need to interact with body tissues without causing inflammation or rejection.

Hypoallergenic: Stainless steel is hypoallergenic, making it suitable for individuals with sensitive skin or allergies to other metals.

Anti-microbial Properties: Hygiene and Safety: Stainless steel's non-porous surface prevents the accumulation of bacteria and other pathogens, which is why it is commonly used in medical instruments and kitchenware. This property ensures a high level of hygiene and reduces the risk of infections.

Traditional Chinese Medicine (TCM):

- Properties: Not traditionally used.
- Modern Uses: Recognized for its durability and resistance to corrosion in modern integrative practices.

Ayurveda:

- Properties: Not traditionally used.
- Modern Uses: Employed for its hypoallergenic properties in contemporary holistic practices.

Holistic Practices:

- Benefits: Durable, hypoallergenic, and used in medical devices and jewelry to support overall health.
- Finger Placement: Worn as needed based on personal preference and skin sensitivity.

PLATINUM

PROPERTIES AND BENEFITS OF PALLADIUM

Palladium is a rare and precious metal known for its catalytic properties and resistance to corrosion. In the context of holistic health and metaphysical practices, palladium is believed to have properties that can support the endocrine system by influencing hormone production and regulation.

Properties of Palladium

> Biocompatibility: Palladium is biocompatible, meaning it does not provoke an immune response when used in medical applications. This makes it suitable for use in various implants and medical devices.

> Catalytic Properties: Palladium acts as a catalyst in chemical reactions, which is believed to support metabolic processes and hormone regulation.

> Stability and Durability: Palladium is highly resistant to corrosion and wear, ensuring its longevity and effectiveness when used in medical devices.

> Antioxidant Effects: Palladium is thought to have antioxidant properties, helping to protect cells from oxidative stress and damage.

Traditional Chinese Medicine (TCM):

- Properties: Not traditionally used.
- Modern Uses: Integrated into modern TCM for its supportive roles in mental clarity and nerve function.

Ayurveda:

- Properties: Not traditionally used.

- Modern Uses: Recognized for its calming and stabilizing properties in contemporary applications.

Holistic Practices:

- Benefits: Enhances mental clarity, reduces stress, and supports nerve function.
- Finger Placement: Often worn on the middle finger for mental clarity and balance.

TITANIUM

PROPERTIES AND BENEFITS OF TITANIUM

Titanium is a strong, lightweight, and corrosion-resistant metal widely used in medical applications, particularly in orthopedic and dental implants. Let's delve into the properties and benefits of titanium, especially in relation to bones and joints.

Properties of Titanium

> Biocompatibility: Titanium is highly biocompatible, meaning the body does not reject it and does not cause adverse reactions when implanted. This makes it ideal for use in medical implants.

> Strength and Durability: Titanium is incredibly strong and durable, providing long-lasting support and stability. It can withstand the mechanical stresses placed on bones and joints.

> Lightweight: Despite its strength, titanium is lightweight, which is beneficial for patients as it reduces the overall weight of implants and makes them more comfortable.

> Corrosion Resistance: Titanium is highly resistant to corrosion, even in the harsh environment of the human body. This ensures the longevity and reliability of titanium implants.

Traditional Chinese Medicine (TCM):

- Properties: Not traditionally used.
- Modern Uses: Used for its biocompatibility and strength in modern medical practices.

Ayurveda:

- Properties: Not traditionally used.
- Modern Uses: Recognized for its supportive role in bone health and strength.

Holistic Practices:

- Benefits: Supports bone health, promotes tissue repair, and enhances overall strength.
- Finger Placement: Commonly worn on the middle finger for structural support.

COBALT

BENEFITS OF COBALT FOR THE URINARY SYSTEM

Kidney Function: Support for Detoxification: Cobalt can support the kidneys in their detoxification processes by activating enzymes involved in metabolizing waste products and toxins.

Reduction of Inflammation: Its anti-inflammatory properties can help alleviate conditions that affect the kidneys, such as nephritis (kidney inflammation).

Bladder Health: Prevention of Infections: The antimicrobial properties of cobalt can help prevent and treat infections in the bladder and urinary tract, reducing the risk of urinary tract infections (UTIs).

Support for Tissue Health: Cobalt can aid in maintaining healthy tissues in the bladder, promoting overall urinary health.

Electrolyte Balance: Cobalt plays a role in maintaining electrolyte balance, which is crucial for proper kidney function and fluid regulation.

Vitamin B12 Production: As a component of vitamin B12, cobalt is essential for producing red blood cells and supporting neurological function, indirectly benefiting the kidneys by ensuring adequate oxygenation and nerve function.

Traditional Chinese Medicine (TCM):

- Properties: Not traditionally used.
- Modern Uses: Used for its supportive role in bone and tissue health in modern integrative practices.

Ayurveda:

- Properties: Not traditionally used.
- Modern Uses: Employed for its strength and healing properties in contemporary holistic practices.

Holistic Practices:

- Benefits: Supports bone health, promotes tissue repair, and enhances strength.
- Finger Placement: Often worn on the middle finger for its core energy and bone support.

NICKEL

PROPERTIES AND BENEFITS OF NICKEL

Nickel is a versatile metal known for its unique properties that make it valuable in various applications, particularly for supporting the muscular system. Here is a detailed overview of the properties of nickel and its benefits for muscular health:

Properties of Nickel

> Durability and Strength: Durability: Nickel is highly durable and can withstand significant wear and tear. This makes it an excellent choice for applications that require long-lasting materials.

> Strength: Nickel's inherent strength contributes to its ability to support and reinforce structures, which is beneficial for muscular health as it can aid in muscle function and recovery.

> Corrosion Resistance: Resistance to Corrosion: Nickel is highly resistant to corrosion, even in harsh environments. This property ensures that nickel remains effective and long-lasting when used in various applications, including those involving bodily contact.

> Magnetic Properties: Magnetism: Nickel is one of the few metals that exhibit magnetic properties. This characteristic can be harnessed in therapeutic practices to influence muscle function and support overall muscular health.

> Hypoallergenic: Biocompatibility: Nickel is generally hypoallergenic and biocompatible, meaning it does not cause adverse reactions when in contact with biological

tissues. This makes it suitable for medical applications and wearable items like jewelry.

Traditional Chinese Medicine (TCM):

- Properties: Not traditionally emphasized.
- Modern Uses: Recognized in contemporary practices for its durability and supportive role in muscle health.

Ayurveda:

- Properties: Not traditionally used.
- Modern Uses: Utilized for its strength and muscle-supporting properties in modern applications.

Holistic Practices:

- Benefits: Enhances muscle strength, supports recovery, and reduces inflammation.
- Finger Placement: Often worn on the thumb for overall strength and on the middle finger for muscular support.

PALLADIUM

PROPERTIES AND BENEFITS OF PALLADIUM

Palladium is a rare and precious metal known for its catalytic properties and resistance to corrosion. In the context of holistic health and metaphysical practices, palladium is believed to have properties that can support various body systems, including the circulatory and immune systems, by influencing hormone production and regulation.

Properties of Palladium

- Biocompatibility: Palladium is biocompatible, meaning it does not provoke an immune response when used in medical applications. This makes it suitable for use in various implants and medical devices.
- Catalytic Properties: Palladium acts as a catalyst in chemical reactions, which is believed to support metabolic processes and hormone regulation.
- Stability and Durability: Palladium is highly resistant to corrosion and wear, ensuring its longevity and effectiveness when used in medical devices.
- Antioxidant Effects: Palladium is thought to have antioxidant properties, helping to protect cells from oxidative stress and damage.

Benefits of Palladium

- Hormone Regulation: Palladium's catalytic properties support the production and regulation of hormones, ensuring optimal functioning of the endocrine glands.
- Metabolic Support: By influencing metabolic processes, palladium can help maintain energy balance and support overall metabolic health.

- Antioxidant Protection: The antioxidant effects of palladium protect cells and tissues from oxidative stress, supporting their health and longevity.
- Stress Response: Palladium is believed to support the adrenal glands, helping the body manage and respond to stress effectively.
- Immune Function: Palladium's biocompatibility and antioxidant properties can enhance immune function, aiding the body's defense against infections and diseases.

Traditional and Holistic Practices

Traditional Chinese Medicine (TCM)

Properties: Palladium is not traditionally used in TCM.

Modern Uses: Integrated into modern TCM for its supportive roles in mental clarity and nerve function.

Ayurveda

Properties: Palladium is not traditionally used in Ayurveda.

Modern Uses: Recognized for its calming and stabilizing properties in contemporary applications.

Holistic Practices

Benefits: Enhances mental clarity, reduces stress, and supports nerve function.

Finger Placement: Often worn on the middle finger for mental clarity and balance.

By understanding the properties and benefits of palladium, individuals can incorporate this metal into their holistic health practices to support various bodily functions and overall well-being.

White vs. Colored Metals: Distributing and Gathering Energy for Holistic Health

The belief that white metals distribute energy and colored metals gather energy is rooted in metaphysical and holistic traditions, which associate different metals with specific energetic properties and effects on the body and mind. Here's an overview of this belief and how it applies to various metals:

WHITE METALS: DISTRIBUTING ENERGY

White metals, such as silver, platinum, and white gold, are thought to have properties that help in the distribution and balancing of energy throughout the body. These metals are often associated with clarity, purity, and cooling effects. Here are some specific beliefs associated with white metals:

Silver:

> Energy Distribution: Silver is believed to distribute energy evenly throughout the body, promoting balance and harmony.

> Cooling Effect: Silver is thought to have cooling properties that can help reduce inflammation and calm the mind.

> Purity and Protection: Silver is often associated with purity and protection, believed to ward off negative energies and enhance overall well-being.

Platinum:

>Clarity and Focus: Platinum is believed to enhance mental clarity and focus, distribute cognitive energy, and support clear thinking.

>Stability: Known for its durability and strength, platinum is thought to bring stability to one's energy, promoting a balanced state.

White Gold:

>Harmonizing: White gold is considered to harmonize energy, providing a balance between the physical and spiritual aspects of life.

>Elevating Vibration: It is believed to elevate one's vibrational frequency, enhancing spiritual growth and awareness.

Stainless Steel:

>Durability and Purity: Stainless steel is known for its hypoallergenic properties and durability, providing a stable and balanced energy.

>Resilience: Associated with resilience and protection, stainless steel can help maintain a steady flow of energy.

Palladium:

>Harmonizing: Balance and Stability: Palladium is considered to harmonize energy, providing a balance between the physical, emotional, and spiritual aspects of life. It promotes a stable and harmonious flow of energy throughout the body.

Elevating Vibration: Enhancing Awareness: Palladium is believed to elevate one's vibrational frequency, enhancing spiritual growth and awareness. It helps individuals connect more deeply with their inner selves and the world around them.

COLORED METALS: GATHERING ENERGY

Colored metals, such as gold, copper, brass, and nickel, are thought to have properties that help gather and focus energy. These metals are often associated with warmth, vitality, and grounding effects. Here are some specific beliefs associated with colored metals:

Gold:

Energy Gathering: Gold is believed to attract and concentrate energy, providing warmth and vitality.

Healing and Regeneration: Gold is thought to promote healing and regeneration, enhancing physical strength and resilience.

Confidence and Success: It is often associated with wealth, success, and confidence, believed to boost one's self-esteem and attract positive outcomes.

Copper:

Conductivity: Copper is known for its excellent conductive properties, thought to enhance the flow of energy and bring it together in a focused manner.

Grounding and Vitality: Copper is believed to ground energy, promoting stability and vitality in the body.

Anti-Inflammatory: Copper is thought to have anti-inflammatory properties, aiding in physical healing and reducing pain.

Brass:

Harmonizing and Balancing: Brass is considered to harmonize and balance energy, bringing together physical and spiritual energies.

Strength and Protection: It is believed to provide strength and protection, enhancing overall resilience and defense against negative influences.

Nickel:

Strength and Vitality: Nickel is associated with enhancing muscle strength and vitality, promoting physical resilience.

Grounding: It is thought to help ground and stabilize energy, supporting overall balance.

Titanium:

Strength and Support: Titanium is known for its strength and biocompatibility, supporting structural integrity and stability.

Healing Properties: Often used in medical applications, titanium is believed to support bone health and overall healing.

Cobalt:

Energy Focusing: Cobalt is believed to concentrate and focus energy, promoting clarity and direction.

Healing and Stability: It is thought to support bone health and tissue repair, enhancing physical stability.

The belief that white metals distribute energy and colored metals gather energy is a part of metaphysical traditions that view metals as having unique energetic properties. White metals like silver and platinum are thought to balance and distribute energy, promoting clarity and harmony, while colored metals like gold and copper are believed to gather and focus energy, providing vitality and grounding. These concepts are applied in various holistic practices to enhance well-being and support overall health.

Chapter 3:
The Five Elements Theory
Basics

The Five Elements and the Human Body

INTRODUCTION TO THE FIVE ELEMENTS THEORY

The Five Elements Theory, also known as Wu Xing, is a fundamental concept in Traditional Chinese Medicine (TCM), philosophy, and cosmology. It describes the dynamic relationships and interactions between different aspects of the natural world and the human body. Understanding this theory provides insight into how TCM practitioners diagnose and treat various health conditions by observing the balance and interplay of these elements.

ORIGINS AND PHILOSOPHICAL FOUNDATIONS

The Five Elements Theory dates back to ancient China, around the 5th century BCE, during the Zhou Dynasty. It was initially used to describe natural phenomena and later integrated into TCM, feng shui, astrology, and other Chinese cultural practices. The theory is rooted in Taoist philosophy, which emphasizes harmony with the Tao (the Way) and balance between Yin and Yang.

THE FIVE ELEMENTS

The five elements in this theory are Fire, Earth, Metal, Water, and Wood. Each element is associated with specific characteristics, bodily organs, emotions, seasons, and more.

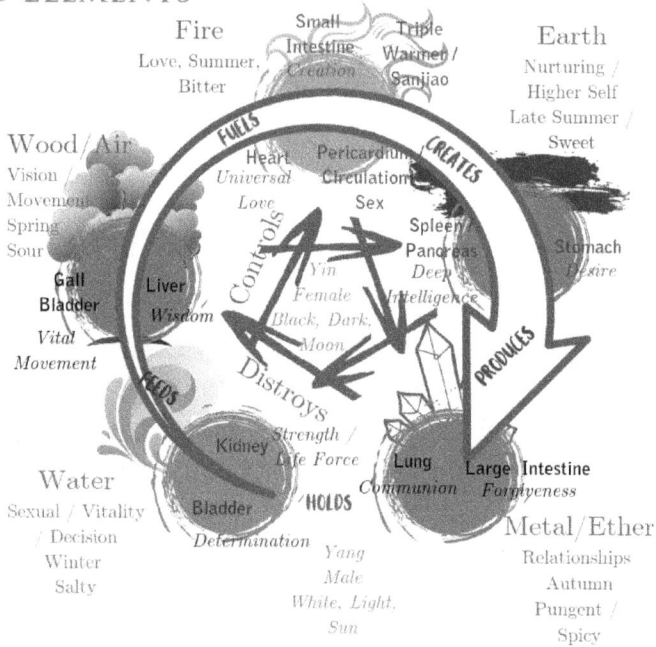

5 ELEMENTS

Fire
Love, Summer,
Bitter

Small Intestine
Triple Warmer / Sanjiao
Creation

Earth
Nurturing /
Higher Self
Late Summer /
Sweet

Wood/Air
Vision /
Movement
Spring
Sour

FUELS
CREATES

Heart
Universal
Love

Pericardium /
Circulation
Sex

Spleen /
Pancreas
Deep
Intelligence

Stomach
Desire

Gall Bladder
Liver
Wisdom

Controls

Yin
Female
Black, Dark,
Moon

Vital
Movement

FEEDS

Distroys

PRODUCES

Kidney
Strength /
Life Force

Lung
Communion

Large Intestine
Forgiveness

Water
Sexual / Vitality
/ Decision
Winter
Salty

Bladder
Determination

HOLDS

Yang
Male
White, Light,
Sun

Metal/Ether
Relationships
Autumn
Pungent /
Spicy

Here's a detailed look at each element:

1. **Fire (Huo)**
   - Characteristics: Heat, intensity, transformation, and activity.
   - Organs: Heart (Yin) and Small Intestine (Yang).
   - Emotions: Joy and excitement.
   - Season: Summer.
   - Direction: South.
   - Color: Red.
   - Sense Organ: Tongue.
   - Tissues: Blood vessels.

- o Examples: Flames, sunlight, and anything that burns and radiates heat.

2. **Earth (Tu)**
   - o Characteristics: Stability, nourishment, and balance.
   - o Organs: Spleen (Yin) and Stomach (Yang).
   - o Emotions: Worry and thoughtfulness.
   - o Season: Late summer.
   - o Direction: Center.
   - o Color: Yellow.
   - o Sense Organ: Mouth.
   - o Tissues: Muscles.
   - o Examples: Soil, mountains, and anything that provides support and nourishment.

3. **Metal (Jin)**
   - o Characteristics: Structure, strength, and refinement.
   - o Organs: Lungs (Yin) and Large Intestine (Yang).
   - o Emotions: Grief and melancholy.
   - o Season: Autumn.
   - o Direction: West.
   - o Color: White.
   - o Sense Organ: Nose.
   - o Tissues: Skin and hair.
   - o Examples: Minerals, rocks, and anything that is solid and structured.

4. **Water (Shui)**
   - o Characteristics: Fluidity, adaptability, and receptiveness.
   - o Organs: Kidneys (Yin) and Urinary Bladder (Yang).
   - o Emotions: Fear and calm.
   - o Season: Winter.
   - o Direction: North.
   - o Color: Blue/black.

- o Sense Organ: Ears.
- o Tissues: Bones.
- o Examples: Rivers, oceans, and anything that flows and nourishes life.

5. **Wood (Mu)**
   - o Characteristics: Growth, expansion, flexibility, and vitality.
   - o Organs: Liver (Yin) and Gall Bladder (Yang).
   - o Emotions: Anger and assertiveness.
   - o Season: Spring.
   - o Direction: East.
   - o Color: Green.
   - o Sense Organ: Eyes.
   - o Tissues: Tendons and ligaments.
   - o Examples: Trees, plants, and anything that grows and expands.
   - o

INTERRELATIONSHIPS BETWEEN THE ELEMENTS

The Five Elements Theory outlines specific relationships and interactions among the elements, which are categorized into generating (sheng) and controlling (ke) cycles:

1. Generating Cycle (Sheng)
   - o Wood generates Fire (wood burns to create fire).
   - o Fire generates Earth (fire's ash enriches the soil).
   - o Earth generates Metal (metal is extracted from the earth).
   - o Metal generates Water (metal condenses water from air).
   - o Water generates Wood (water nourishes plants).

2. Controlling Cycle (Ke)
   o Wood controls Earth (roots penetrate and stabilize soil).
   o Earth controls Water (earth dams and absorbs water).
   o Water controls Fire (water extinguishes fire).
   o Fire controls Metal (fire melts metal).
   o Metal controls Wood (metal tools cut wood).

APPLICATION IN TRADITIONAL CHINESE MEDICINE

In TCM, the balance and harmony between the five elements are crucial for health and well-being. Imbalances or disruptions in the elements' relationships can lead to illness. TCM practitioners use the Five Elements Theory to:

Diagnose: Identify imbalances by observing symptoms and correlating them with the elements.

Treat: Use acupuncture, herbal medicine, diet, and lifestyle changes to restore balance among the elements.

Example Applications

Liver (Wood) Imbalance: Symptoms might include anger, irritability, and eye problems. Treatment could involve herbs that soothe the liver and dietary changes to support Wood.

Heart (Fire) Imbalance: Symptoms might include insomnia, anxiety, and tongue issues. Treatment could include acupuncture points that calm the heart and herbs that balance Fire.

The Five Elements Theory provides a comprehensive framework for understanding the intricate relationships within the human body and the natural world. It emphasizes the importance of balance and harmony in maintaining health, guiding TCM practitioners in diagnosing and treating various conditions. This ancient wisdom continues to be relevant, offering valuable insights into holistic health and well-being.

How Elements Correspond to Body Systems

In Traditional Chinese Medicine (TCM), the Five Elements Theory links each element to specific organs, tissues, emotions, and physiological processes. This holistic view helps practitioners diagnose and treat various health conditions by observing imbalances in these relationships. Here's a detailed look at how each element corresponds to different body systems:

1. Wood Element

Associated Organs:

- o Liver (Yin Organ): The liver is responsible for storing blood and ensuring the smooth flow of Qi (energy) throughout the body. It influences emotional stability and eye health.
- o Gall Bladder (Yang Organ): The gall bladder stores and excretes bile, aiding in digestion and decision-making processes.

Associated Body Systems:

- o Musculoskeletal System: Wood governs the health of tendons and ligaments, which are critical for movement and flexibility.
- o Nervous System: It influences the autonomic nervous system, affecting stress response and emotional regulation.

Emotions:

- ○ Positive: Creativity, assertiveness, and growth.
- ○ Negative: Anger, frustration, and irritability.

2. Fire Element

Associated Organs:

- ○ Heart (Yin Organ): The heart governs blood circulation and houses the Shen (mind or spirit), influencing mental clarity and emotional well-being.
- ○ Small Intestine (Yang Organ): The small intestine is involved in nutrient absorption and sorting pure from impure substances.

Associated Body Systems:

- ○ Circulatory System: Fire governs the health of blood vessels and the overall circulatory system, ensuring proper blood flow and cardiovascular health.
- ○ Nervous System: It also plays a role in the central nervous system, affecting mental function and consciousness.

Emotions:

- ○ Positive: Joy, enthusiasm, and passion.
- ○ Negative: Anxiety, restlessness, and overexcitement.

3. Earth Element

Associated Organs:

- ○ Spleen (Yin Organ): The spleen is crucial for digestion and transforming food into Qi and blood. It also manages blood containment and fluid balance.

- o Stomach (Yang Organ): The stomach is responsible for receiving and breaking down food, playing a key role in digestion.

Associated Body Systems:

- o Digestive System: Earth governs the gastrointestinal tract, influencing digestion, nutrient absorption, and metabolism.
- o Muscular System: It also affects muscle tone and strength.

Emotions:

- o Positive: Compassion, nurturing, and stability.
- o Negative: Worry, overthinking, and pensiveness.

4. Metal Element

Associated Organs:

- o Lungs (Yin Organ): The lungs are responsible for respiration, regulating Qi, and protecting against external pathogens. They also influence the skin and body hair.
- o Large Intestine (Yang Organ): The large intestine handles the final stage of digestion, absorbing water and excreting waste.

Associated Body Systems:

- o Respiratory System: Metal governs the health of the lungs and respiratory tract, ensuring efficient breathing and oxygen exchange.
- o Integumentary System: It also influences skin health, including its ability to protect and regulate temperature.

Emotions:

- o Positive: Grief, reflection, and detachment.
- o Negative: Sadness, melancholy, and rigidity.

5. Water Element

Associated Organs:

- o Kidneys (Yin Organ): The kidneys store essence (Jing), regulate water metabolism, and influence growth, development, and reproduction.
- o Urinary Bladder (Yang Organ): The bladder stores and excretes urine, playing a role in fluid regulation.

Associated Body Systems:

- o Urinary System: Water governs the kidneys and bladder, influencing fluid balance, detoxification, and waste elimination.
- o Endocrine System: It also affects hormonal balance and reproductive health.

Emotions:

- o Positive: Fear, calmness, and willpower.
- o Negative: Fear, insecurity, and anxiety.

PRACTICAL APPLICATIONS IN TCM
Diagnosis:

Practitioners assess symptoms and correlate them with the Five Elements. For instance, liver imbalances (Wood) may manifest as eye problems, anger, or muscle stiffness.

Treatment:

> Acupuncture: Specific points along the meridians corresponding to each element are stimulated to restore balance.

> Herbal Medicine: Herbs are prescribed to strengthen or calm particular elements. For example, cooling herbs might be used to calm excessive Fire.

Lifestyle Recommendations:

> Diet, exercise, and stress management techniques are tailored to support the balance of the Five Elements. For example, sour foods are recommended to support the liver (Wood), while bitter foods may be suggested to calm the heart (Fire).

The Five Elements Theory offers a comprehensive framework for understanding the interplay between different body systems and their corresponding elements. By recognizing these relationships, TCM practitioners can provide holistic and personalized care that addresses both physical and emotional health.

THE FIVE ELEMENTS IN AYURVEDA

Ayurveda incorporates the concept of elements, though there are some differences from Traditional Chinese Medicine (TCM). Both systems recognize the importance of elemental balance in maintaining health, but they have distinct interpretations and applications of these elements.

In Ayurveda, the concept of elements is fundamental, and it recognizes five basic elements, or "Panchamahabhutas":

1. **Earth (Prithvi):** Represents solidity and stability. It is associated with the physical structure of the body, including bones and tissues.
2. **Water (Jala or Apas):** Represents fluidity and cohesiveness. It is associated with bodily fluids like blood, lymph, and digestive juices.
3. **Fire (Agni):** Represents transformation and metabolism. It is associated with digestive and metabolic processes.
4. **Air (Vayu):** Represents movement and transportation. It is associated with the nervous system and the movement of bodily functions.
5. **Ether (Akasha):** Represents space and expansiveness. It is associated with cavities and channels within the body, such as the mouth and digestive tract.

KEY DIFFERENCES BETWEEN AYURVEDA AND TCM ELEMENTS
Number of Elements:

Ayurveda includes Ether (Akasha) as one of its five elements, while TCM includes Metal (Jin).

TCM does not include Ether but instead incorporates Metal, which is not a separate element in Ayurveda.

Elemental Associations:

In Ayurveda, elements form the basis of the three Doshas (Vata, Pitta, and Kapha), which are fundamental bodily bio-energies.

> Vata (Air and Ether): Governs movement and is associated with the nervous system.

> Pitta (Fire and Water): Governs digestion and metabolism.

> Kapha (Earth and Water): Governs structure and cohesion.

In TCM, the Five Elements correspond to specific organs, emotions, seasons, and various physiological processes without forming triadic groups like the Doshas in Ayurveda.

PHILOSOPHICAL APPROACH:

> Ayurveda: Focuses on individual constitution (Prakriti) and aims to maintain balance according to one's unique doshic makeup. It involves personalized dietary, lifestyle, and herbal recommendations to balance the elements within an individual's constitution.

> TCM: Focuses on the balance and flow of Qi (energy) through the body's meridians and the interactions among the Five Elements. Treatments often involve acupuncture, herbal medicine, and exercises like Tai Chi or Qigong to balance Qi and the elements.

DIAGNOSTIC METHODS:

> Ayurveda: Diagnosis is based on the assessment of Dosha imbalances through pulse reading, tongue examination, and understanding an individual's Prakriti.

TCM: Diagnosis involves observing signs and symptoms related to the Five Elements, pulse diagnosis, tongue examination, and understanding the flow of Qi.

While Ayurveda and TCM emphasize the balance of natural elements within the body to maintain health, they differ in their classification and application of these elements. Ayurveda's approach is more centered around the three Doshas derived from the five elements, whereas TCM directly links the Five Elements to specific organs and their functions. These distinctions highlight the unique philosophies and methodologies that each system employs to achieve holistic health and wellness.

Chapter 4:
Fingers of the Hand

Each finger on the human hand has a specific name, both in common parlance and in anatomical terminology:

- Thumb (Pollex):
  - Common Name: Thumb
  - Anatomical Name: Pollex
- Index Finger (Second Digit):
  - Common Name: Index Finger, Pointer Finger, Forefinger
  - Anatomical Name: Digitus Secundus, Digitus II
- Middle Finger (Third Digit):
  - Common Name: Middle Finger
  - Anatomical Name: Digitus Medius, Digitus III
- Ring Finger (Fourth Digit):
  - Common Name: Ring Finger
  - Anatomical Name: Digitus Annularis, Digitus IV
- Little Finger (Fifth Digit):
  - Common Name: Little Finger, Pinky Finger
  - Anatomical Name: Digitus Minimus, Digitus V

These names are widely used in everyday language and medical contexts to refer to the fingers of the hand.

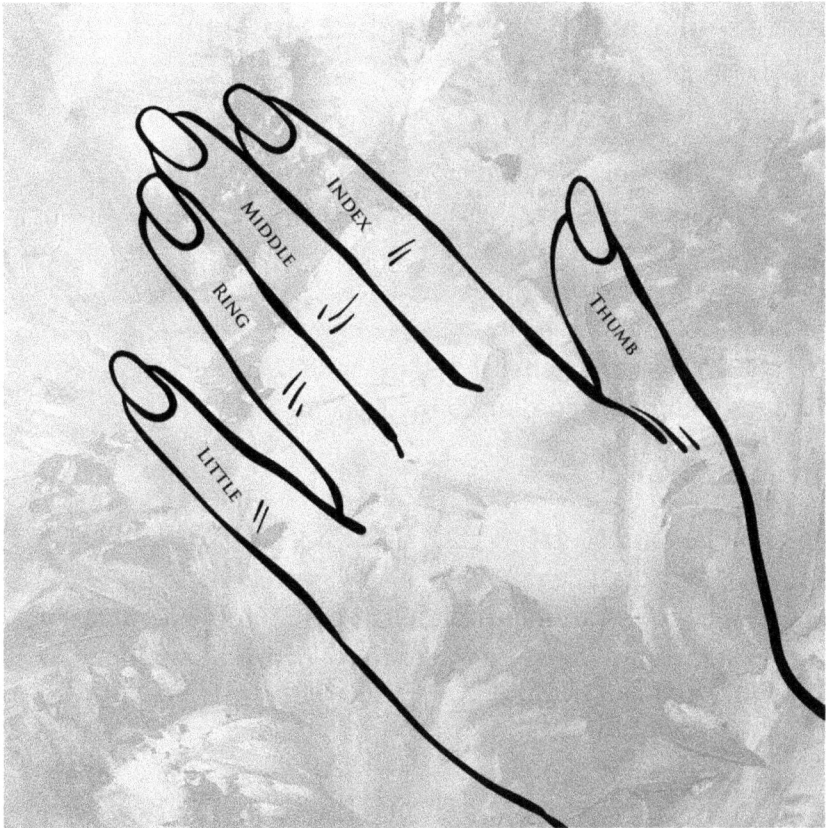

Finger-Element Correspondences in Traditional Chinese Medicine (TCM)

In Traditional Chinese Medicine (TCM), the Five Elements Theory (Wood, Fire, Earth, Metal, Water) is applied in various ways to understand how different body parts and natural phenomena are interconnected. Each finger can correspond to a specific element, which relates to certain organs and functions. Here is a general outline of which finger corresponds to each element according to the Five Elements Theory:

Thumb (Metal)

- o Element: Metal
- o Associated Organs: Lungs and Large Intestine
- o Functions: Metal is related to respiratory and digestive functions. It also represents the ability to eliminate waste and maintain structure and form.

Index Finger (Water)

- o Element: Water
- o Associated Organs: Kidneys and Bladder
- o Functions: Water governs fluid balance, reproductive health, and the body's ability to store and conserve energy.

Middle Finger (Fire)

- o Element: Fire
- o Associated Organs: Heart and Small Intestine
- o Functions: Fire relates to circulatory and digestive functions, emotional stability, and mental clarity. It governs warmth and vitality in the body.

Ring Finger (Earth)

- o Element: Earth
- o Associated Organs: Spleen and Stomach
- o Functions: Earth is associated with digestion, nourishment, and transformation of food into energy. It represents stability and support.

Little Finger (Wood)

- o Element: Wood
- o Associated Organs: Liver and Gall Bladder

Functions: Wood governs growth, flexibility, and the smooth flow of energy throughout the body. It is related to detoxification and emotional regulation.

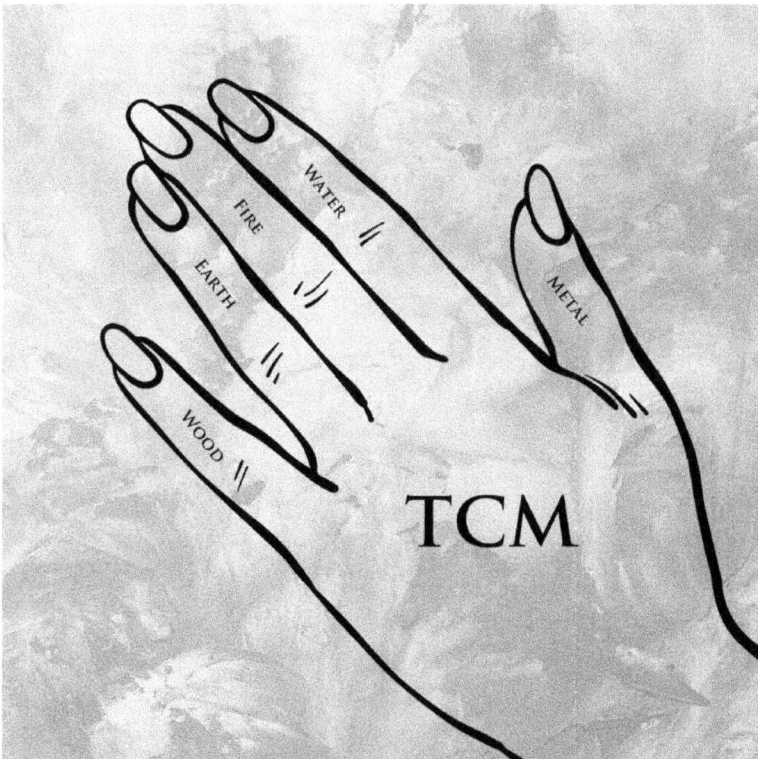

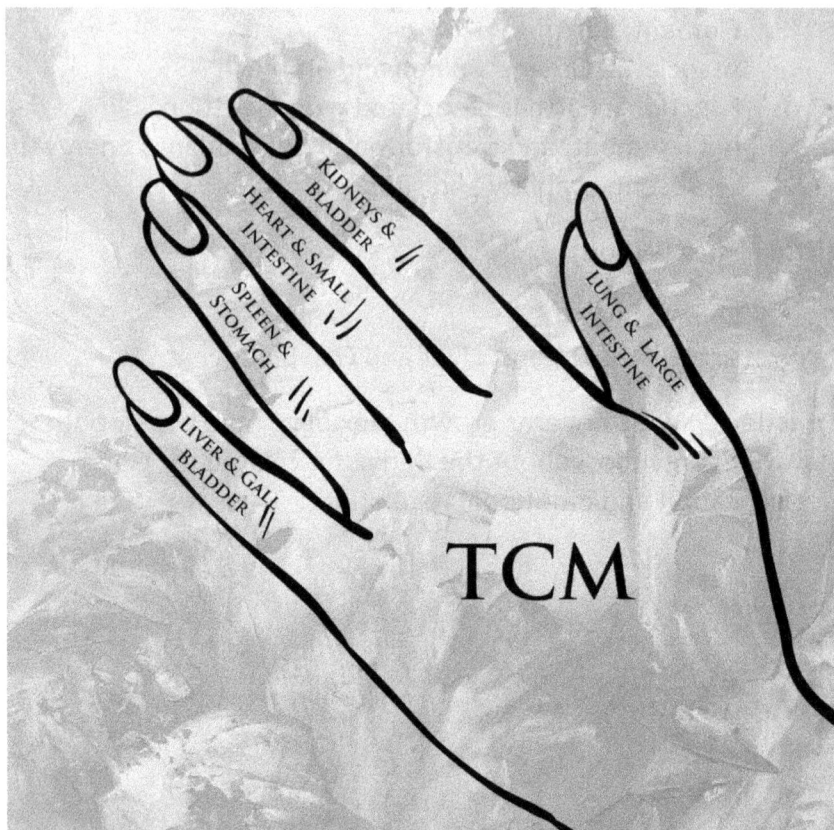

TCM DETAILED CORRESPONDENCES AND ROLES:
Thumb (Metal)

- o Associated Meridians: Lung Meridian, Large Intestine Meridian
- o Emotional Aspect: Grief and letting go
- o Season: Autumn
- o Color: White
- o Taste: Pungent

Index Finger (Water)

- o Associated Meridians: Kidney Meridian, Bladder Meridian
- o Emotional Aspect: Fear and courage
- o Season: Winter
- o Color: Blue/Black
- o Taste: Salty

Middle Finger (Fire)

- o Associated Meridians: Heart Meridian, Small Intestine Meridian
- o Emotional Aspect: Joy and love
- o Season: Summer
- o Color: Red
- o Taste: Bitter

Ring Finger (Earth)

- o Associated Meridians: Spleen Meridian, Stomach Meridian
- o Emotional Aspect: Worry and nurturing
- o Season: Late Summer
- o Color: Yellow
- o Taste: Sweet

Little Finger (Wood)

- o Associated Meridians: Liver Meridian, Gall Bladder Meridian
- o Emotional Aspect: Anger and kindness
- o Season: Spring
- o Color: Green
- o Taste: Sour

INTEGRATION WITH HEALING PRACTICES

- o **Acupuncture and Acupressure**: Practitioners may stimulate specific points on the fingers to influence the corresponding organs and balance the Five Elements.
- o **Wearing Rings**: Some traditions suggest wearing rings made of certain metals on specific fingers to enhance the corresponding element's energy and support related bodily functions.
- o **Mudras**: Hand gestures used in yoga and meditation can also align with these correspondences to promote balance and health.

Finger-Element Correspondences in Ayurveda

In Ayurveda, the Five Elements (Pancha Mahabhutas) are fundamental to understanding how different parts of the body and natural phenomena are interconnected. Each finger can correspond to a specific element, which relates to certain organs and functions. Here is a general outline of which finger corresponds to each element according to Ayurvedic principles:

Thumb (Fire)

- o Element: Fire (Agni)
- o Associated Organs: Stomach and Liver
- o Functions: Fire is related to metabolism, digestion, and transformation. It governs the body's ability to process food and convert it into energy.

Index Finger (Air)

- o Element: Air (Vayu)
- o Associated Organs: Lungs and Large Intestine
- o Functions: Air governs movement, respiration, and communication. It is responsible for the flow of breath and the elimination of waste.

Middle Finger (Ether)

- o Element: Ether (Akasha)
- o Associated Organs: Heart and Small Intestine
- o Functions: Ether represents space and the mind. It governs mental clarity, consciousness, and the space within the body where all other elements interact.

Ring Finger (Earth)

- o Element: Earth (Prithvi)
- o Associated Organs: Spleen and Stomach
- o Functions: Earth is associated with stability, structure, and nourishment. It represents the physical body and the tissues.

Little Finger (Water)

- o Element: Water (Jala)
- o Associated Organs: Kidneys and Bladder

Functions: Water governs fluid balance, hydration, and the body's ability to cleanse and detoxify.

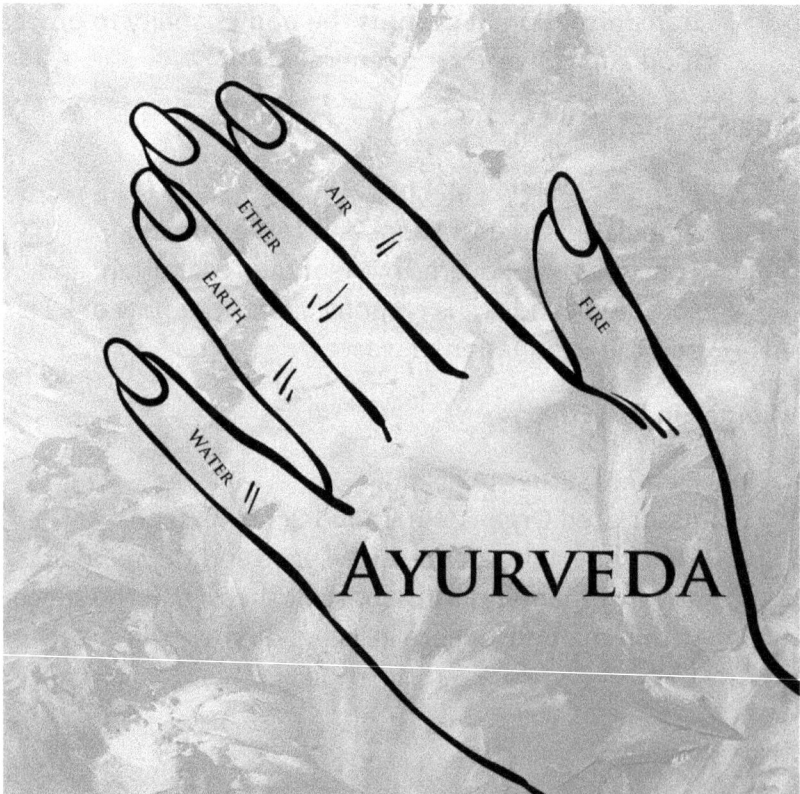

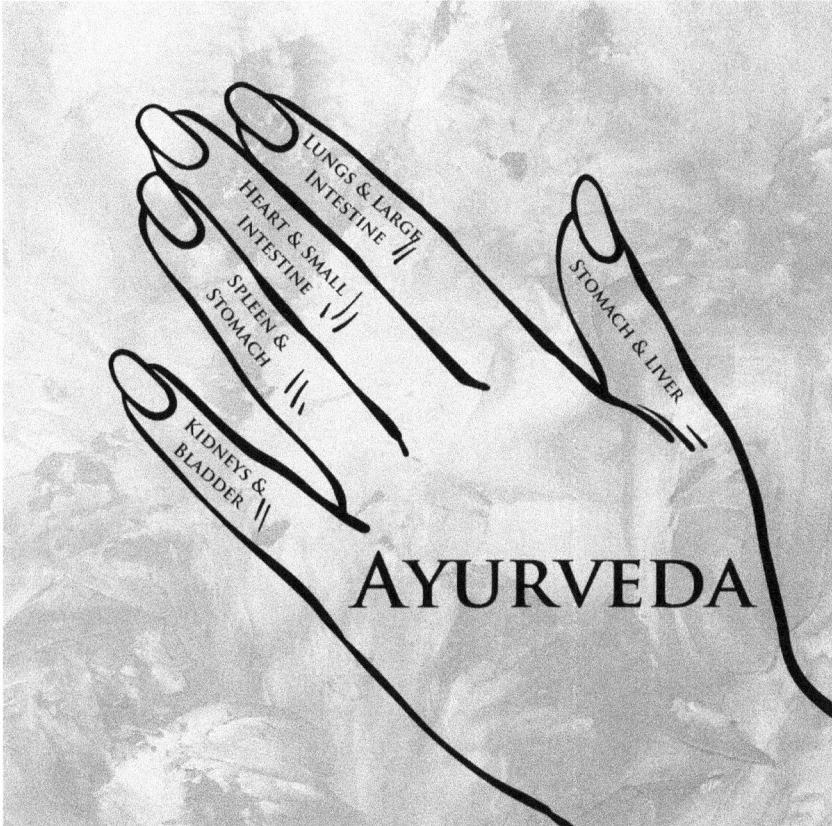

LUNGS & LARGE INTESTINE
HEART & SMALL INTESTINE
SPLEEN & STOMACH
STOMACH & LIVER
KIDNEYS & BLADDER

AYURVEDA

DETAILED CORRESPONDENCES AND ROLES:
Thumb (Fire)

- o Associated Dosha: Pitta
- o Emotional Aspect: Courage and determination
- o Season: Summer
- o Color: Red
- o Taste: Pungent
- o Functions: Balances digestion and metabolism, promotes warmth and vitality.

Index Finger (Air)

- o Associated Dosha: Vata
- o Emotional Aspect: Movement and creativity
- o Season: Autumn
- o Color: Blue
- o Taste: Bitter
- o Functions: Regulates breath and elimination, enhances movement and flexibility.

Middle Finger (Ether)

- o Associated Dosha: Vata
- o Emotional Aspect: Mental clarity and intuition
- o Season: Winter
- o Color: Black
- o Taste: Astringent
- o Functions: Enhances mental clarity and consciousness, governs the space within the body.

Ring Finger (Earth)

- o Associated Dosha: Kapha
- o Emotional Aspect: Stability and nurturing
- o Season: Spring
- o Color: Yellow
- o Taste: Sweet
- o Functions: Provides structure and stability, supports physical strength and endurance.

Little Finger (Water)

- o Associated Dosha: Kapha
- o Emotional Aspect: Calmness and compassion
- o Season: Late Winter/Early Spring
- o Color: White
- o Taste: Salty

    o   Functions: Maintains fluid balance and hydration, promotes detoxification and cleansing.

INTEGRATION WITH HEALING PRACTICES
Mudras (Hand Gestures)

> Usage: Mudras can align with these correspondences to promote balance and health by channeling the energy of the elements through specific hand gestures.

> Examples:

> Agni Mudra: Involves the thumb and balances the fire element, enhancing digestion and metabolism.

> Vayu Mudra: Involves the index finger and balances the air element, improving respiration and reducing anxiety.

Ayurvedic Treatments

> Diet and Lifestyle: Specific foods, herbs, and practices can balance the corresponding elements associated with each finger.

> Massage and Oils: Using specific oils and massage techniques on the fingers can help balance the doshas and elements.

Yoga and Pranayama

> Yoga Poses: Certain yoga poses can activate the corresponding elements and doshas associated with each finger.

> Breathing Exercises: Pranayama practices can enhance the flow of prana (life force) through the elements represented by the fingers.

By understanding the finger-element correspondences in Ayurveda, practitioners can use various techniques, including mudras, dietary adjustments, and yoga practices, to balance the body's elements and promote overall health and well-being. This holistic approach integrates physical, mental, and emotional aspects to create harmony and balance in life.

Ayurveda Mudras: Hand Gestures for Balance and Health

Mudras are symbolic hand gestures used in yoga and meditation practices to channel and balance the body's energy. These gestures are believed to influence the flow of prana (life force) and affect various aspects of physical and mental health. Each mudra is associated with specific elements and corresponding fingers, aligning with the principles of the Five Elements Theory.

BENEFITS OF MUDRAS

Balancing Energy: Mudras help balance the five elements within the body, promoting overall health and well-being.

Mental Clarity: Regular practice can improve concentration, reduce stress, and enhance mental clarity.

Physical Health: Specific mudras target different organs and systems, supporting respiratory, digestive, cardiovascular, and immune health.

Emotional Stability: Mudras can help regulate emotions, promoting a sense of calm and balance.

How to Practice Mudras
Steps:

1. Find a Quiet Place: Sit comfortably in a quiet place where you won't be disturbed.
2. Relax Your Body: Take a few deep breaths to relax your body and mind.
3. Form the Mudra: Use both hands to form the desired mudra, maintaining gentle pressure between the fingertips.
4. Focus on Your Breath: Close your eyes and focus on your breath, directing your attention to the area of the body associated with the mudra.
5. Meditate: Hold the mudra for at least 5 to 15 minutes. You can extend this time as you become more comfortable with the practice.

Here's a detailed look at how mudras can align with finger-organ correspondences to promote balance and health:

The Five Elements and Corresponding Mudras
1. Thumb (Fire)

Mudra: Agni Mudra (Fire Mudra)

Gesture: Bend the ring finger and press it down with the thumb, while keeping the other fingers extended.

Benefits: Increases the fire element in the body, boosting metabolism, digestion, and energy levels. It is also useful for weight management and improving eyesight.

Applications: Enhances cardiovascular health and boosts energy, aiding in conditions like fatigue and poor circulation.

2. Index Finger (Air)

Mudra: Vayu Mudra (Air Mudra)

Gesture: Fold the index finger to touch the base of the thumb, and press the thumb over it, while keeping the other fingers extended.

Benefits: Balances the air element, improving conditions related to air imbalance such as anxiety, stress, and nervous disorders.

Applications: Helps manage anxiety, stress, and related respiratory conditions.

3. Middle Finger (Ether/Space)

Mudra: Akasha Mudra (Space Mudra)

Gesture: Touch the tip of the middle finger to the tip of the thumb, while keeping the other fingers extended.

Benefits: Increases the ether element in the body, promoting a sense of openness and space. It aids in detoxification and mental clarity.

Applications: Supports mental clarity and helps with detoxification processes.

4. Ring Finger (Earth)

Mudra: Prithvi Mudra (Earth Mudra)

Gesture: Touch the tip of the ring finger to the tip of the thumb, while keeping the other fingers extended.

Benefits: Balances the earth element in the body, promoting strength, stability, and grounding. It enhances physical health and vitality.

Applications: Useful for improving strength, stability, and overall physical health.

5. Little Finger (Water)

Mudra: Varuna Mudra (Water Mudra)

Gesture: Touch the tip of the little finger to the tip of the thumb, while keeping the other fingers extended.

Benefits: Balances the water element, improving fluid regulation and circulation. It helps with hydration, skin conditions, and kidney health.

Applications: Supports kidney function and helps manage conditions related to fluid imbalance.

Alternative Element Correspondences:

In some traditions, the elements may correspond differently to the fingers:

For the Little Finger (Ether)

Mudra: Jnana Mudra (Knowledge Mudra) or Chin Mudra (Consciousness Mudra)

Gesture: Touch the tip of the index finger to the tip of the thumb, while keeping the other fingers extended.

Benefits: Enhances concentration, memory, and mental clarity.

Applications: Helps in managing stress and promoting mental clarity, supporting overall cognitive health.

Chapter 5:
Body Systems

Body Systems

The human body comprises several systems that work together to maintain overall health and function. Here are the primary systems of the body:

- **Circulatory System**: Includes the heart, blood, and blood vessels. It transports nutrients, oxygen, and hormones to cells and removes waste products.
- **Respiratory System**: Consists of the lungs and airways. It facilitates the exchange of oxygen and carbon dioxide between the body and the environment.
- **Digestive System**: Includes the mouth, esophagus, stomach, intestines, liver, pancreas, and gallbladder. It breaks down food, absorbs nutrients, and eliminates waste.
- **Nervous System**: Comprises the brain, spinal cord, and peripheral nerves. It controls and coordinates body activities by transmitting signals between different body parts.
- **Skeletal System**: Comprises the bones, tendons, ligaments, and joints. It provides the structural framework for the body, shields internal organs from damage, stores essential minerals, such as calcium and phosphorus, and produces blood cells in the bone marrow.

- **Immune System**: Though often considered part of the lymphatic system, it includes cells, tissues, and organs that work together to defend the body against pathogens.
- **Integumentary System**: Consists of the skin, hair, nails, and exocrine glands. It protects the body from external damage, regulates temperature, and provides sensory information.
- **Reproductive System**: In females, it includes the ovaries, fallopian tubes, uterus, and vagina. In males, it includes the testes, vas deferens, prostate, and penis. It is responsible for producing offspring.
- **Endocrine System**: Includes glands such as the pituitary, thyroid, adrenal, and pancreas. It produces hormones that regulate metabolism, growth, reproduction, and other functions.
- **Urinary System**: Includes the kidneys, ureters, bladder, and urethra. It removes waste products from the blood and maintains fluid and electrolyte balance.
- **Muscular System**: Consists of muscles, tendons, and ligaments. It facilitates movement by contracting and pulling on bones and Generates heat through muscle activity to help maintain body temperature.
- **Lymphatic System**: Comprises lymph nodes and lymphatic vessels. It defends against infections and maintains fluid balance.

Each of these systems plays a crucial role in maintaining the body's homeostasis and overall health.

Chapter 6:
The Circulatory System

Overview of the Circulatory System

The circulatory system, also known as the cardiovascular system, is responsible for the transportation of blood, nutrients, oxygen, carbon dioxide, and hormones throughout the body. It consists of the heart, blood vessels (arteries, veins, and capillaries), and blood. The primary functions of the circulatory system include:

- **Transportation:** Delivering oxygen and nutrients to cells and removing waste products.
- **Regulation:** Maintaining body temperature, pH balance, and fluid balance.
- **Protection:** Defending against infections and blood loss through clotting mechanisms.

METAL TO BALANCE THE CIRCULATORY SYSTEM
GOLD: THE HEART AND BLOOD VESSELS
COPPER: THE HEART AND BLOOD VESSELS

BENEFITS OF GOLD FOR THE CIRCULATORY SYSTEM:

Enhanced Blood Circulation: Gold is believed to promote better blood flow and circulation, supporting the heart and blood vessels.

Heart Health: Wearing gold is thought to strengthen the heart and improve cardiac function, making it beneficial for overall heart health.

Emotional Stability: Gold is linked to emotional stability and balance, which can reduce stress and indirectly support heart health by promoting a sense of calm.

Anti-inflammatory Effects: The anti-inflammatory properties of gold can help reduce inflammation in blood vessels, potentially lowering the risk of cardiovascular diseases.

BENEFITS OF COPPER FOR THE CIRCULATORY SYSTEM:

Enhanced Blood Flow: Copper is believed to support healthy blood flow and circulation, which is essential for maintaining cardiovascular health.

Reduces Inflammation: Copper's anti-inflammatory properties help reduce inflammation in the blood vessels, supporting overall vascular health.

Supports Red Blood Cell Formation: Copper is essential in the formation of hemoglobin and red blood cells, crucial for transporting oxygen throughout the body.

Antimicrobial Protection:

Copper's antimicrobial properties can help prevent infections that may affect the circulatory system, promoting overall cardiovascular health.

Vascular Health: Copper contributes to the structural integrity and elasticity of blood vessels, supporting the overall function of the circulatory system.

SAFETY AND CONSIDERATIONS FOR GOLD AND COPPER AND THE CIRCULATORY SYSTEM

GOLD
Safety and Considerations:

Allergic Reactions: While rare, some individuals may be allergic to gold. Symptoms can include skin irritation, rashes, or itching where the gold makes contact with the skin. It is essential to monitor for any signs of an allergic reaction and discontinue use if symptoms occur.

Quality and Purity: Ensure that the gold used in rings and other jewelry is of high quality and free from harmful contaminants. Pure gold (24 karat) is often too soft for practical use, so it is alloyed with other metals, which can sometimes cause allergic reactions or reduce its beneficial properties.

Proper Usage: Wearing gold rings should complement, not replace, conventional medical treatments for circulatory issues. It is crucial to use gold as a supportive measure alongside professional medical advice.

Long-Term Use: Regularly assess the condition of gold jewelry for any signs of wear and tear. Damaged rings can cause skin irritation or reduce the effectiveness of their beneficial properties.

Emotional Impact: While gold is often associated with emotional stability and balance, it is essential to be mindful of its potential psychological effects. If wearing gold seems to cause emotional distress or imbalance, consider reassessing its use and placement.

COPPER

Safety and Considerations:

Skin Reactions: Copper can cause skin reactions in some individuals, including green discoloration or irritation where the copper contacts the skin. These reactions are usually harmless but can be aesthetically undesirable. Monitoring for any adverse reactions and adjusting usage as necessary is important.

Copper Toxicity: Excessive exposure to copper can lead to copper toxicity, characterized by symptoms such as nausea, vomiting, abdominal pain, and liver damage. It is crucial to ensure that copper exposure remains within safe limits, especially if using multiple copper items or supplements.

Quality and Purity: Ensure that the copper used in rings and other jewelry is of high quality and free from harmful contaminants. Impure copper can contain traces of other metals that may cause adverse reactions or reduce its beneficial properties.

Proper Usage: Copper rings should be used as a supportive measure alongside conventional medical treatments for circulatory issues. Consult with a healthcare professional before incorporating copper into your health regimen, especially if you have existing health conditions.

Cleaning and Maintenance: Regularly clean copper jewelry to prevent the buildup of dirt and oils, which can reduce its effectiveness and cause skin reactions. Proper maintenance ensures the longevity and safety of copper rings.

Interactions with Other Metals: Be mindful of wearing copper alongside other metals. Certain combinations may cause skin reactions or reduce the effectiveness of the metals' beneficial properties. It is essential to test and monitor the effects of wearing multiple metal rings.

Traditional Uses of Gold in Circulatory Health

Gold has been valued not only for its beauty and rarity but also for its therapeutic properties throughout history. Various cultures have utilized gold in traditional medicine to promote circulatory health and treat related ailments. Here are some of the traditional uses of gold in circulatory health:

1. Ayurveda

Swarna Bhasma:

Description: Swarna Bhasma is a traditional Ayurvedic preparation of gold ash. It is made by purifying and calcining gold through a complex process to produce a fine, bioavailable powder.

Uses in Circulatory Health:

Heart Tonic: Swarna Bhasma is believed to strengthen the heart and improve cardiac function.

Blood Circulation: It is used to enhance blood circulation and support the overall cardiovascular system.

Vitality and Longevity: Regular use of Swarna Bhasma is said to promote longevity and vitality, contributing to a healthy circulatory system.

2. Traditional Chinese Medicine (TCM)

Gold in Acupuncture:

Description: Gold needles are sometimes used in acupuncture to stimulate specific points on the body.

Uses in Circulatory Health:

Yang Tonification: Gold is associated with the Yang energy, which is believed to support heart function and improve circulation.

Qi Flow: Using gold needles in acupuncture is thought to enhance the flow of Qi (vital energy) throughout the body, ensuring the smooth functioning of the circulatory system.

Herbal Formulations:

Description: Gold has been included in certain herbal formulations in TCM.

Uses in Circulatory Health:

Heart and Blood Vessels: Formulations containing gold are used to tonify the heart and support the health of blood vessels.

3. Ancient Egypt

Gold for Royalty:

Description: Gold was considered the flesh of the gods and was used extensively in rituals and as offerings.

Uses in Circulatory Health:

Spiritual and Physical Health: Pharaohs and nobility wore gold not just as a symbol of wealth but also for its believed ability to promote physical health, including the heart and circulation.

4. Medieval Alchemy

Elixirs and Potions:

Description: Alchemists sought to create the Elixir of Life, which often included gold.

Uses in Circulatory Health:

Purification and Longevity: Gold was believed to purify the body and soul, enhancing blood circulation and overall vitality.

Health and Immortality: Alchemical texts suggest that consuming gold-based elixirs could improve health and potentially grant immortality.

ANECDOTAL AND HISTORICAL EVIDENCE
Personal Accounts:

Vitality and Energy: Historical texts and personal accounts from various cultures describe gold as a metal that boosts energy levels and overall vitality, which indirectly supports circulatory health.

Emotional Stability: Wearing gold jewelry is believed to calm the mind and reduce stress, which can positively affect heart health and circulation.

The traditional uses of gold in circulatory health span various cultures and practices, from Ayurvedic and TCM preparations to ancient Egyptian rituals and medieval alchemy. These practices highlight gold's perceived ability to strengthen the heart, enhance blood circulation, and promote overall vitality and longevity. While these traditional uses provide valuable insights, modern scientific research continues to explore and validate these ancient beliefs.

Modern Applications and Case Studies

Gold continues to play a significant role in modern medicine, particularly in the treatment of cardiovascular conditions and in advanced therapeutic technologies. Here's an overview of contemporary applications and notable case studies that highlight gold's relevance in circulatory health:

1. Medical Implants and Devices

Stents and Pacemakers:

Usage: Gold is used in the construction of stents and pacemakers due to its biocompatibility and resistance to corrosion. These devices are crucial for maintaining open blood vessels and regulating heart rhythms.

Benefits: Gold-coated stents reduce the risk of restenosis (re-narrowing of the artery) and improve the longevity of the device. Gold's conductivity is also beneficial in ensuring the reliable functioning of pacemakers.

2. Gold Nanoparticles in Drug Delivery

Targeted Drug Delivery:

Usage: Gold nanoparticles (AuNPs) are increasingly used in targeted drug delivery systems. These nanoparticles can be designed to attach to specific cells or tissues, delivering drugs directly to the affected areas.

Benefits: This targeted approach reduces side effects and increases the efficacy of treatments, particularly in cancer and cardiovascular therapies.

Case Study: A study published in the Journal of Nanobiotechnology demonstrated the effectiveness of gold nanoparticles in delivering anti-cancer drugs to tumor sites with minimal side effects (Journal of Nanobiotechnology).

Cardiovascular Applications:

Usage: Gold nanoparticles are used to deliver drugs that can dissolve arterial plaques or prevent clot formation, directly targeting problematic areas in the cardiovascular system.

Case Study: Research published in the Journal of the American College of Cardiology highlighted the use of gold nanoparticles to improve drug delivery for treating atherosclerosis. The study showed that gold nanoparticles could be used to deliver anti-inflammatory drugs directly to arterial plaques, reducing inflammation and stabilizing the plaques.

3. Anti-inflammatory Properties

Rheumatoid Arthritis Treatment:

Usage: Gold salts (such as aurothiomalate) have been used for decades to treat rheumatoid arthritis due to their anti-inflammatory properties.

Benefits: These compounds help reduce joint inflammation and pain, indirectly benefiting circulatory health by reducing overall systemic inflammation.

Case Study: Clinical trials and long-term studies have documented the effectiveness of gold salts in reducing symptoms and slowing the progression of rheumatoid arthritis.

4. Diagnostic and Imaging Tools

Gold Nanoparticles in Imaging:

Usage: Gold nanoparticles are used in various imaging techniques, such as computed tomography (CT) scans and photoacoustic imaging, to enhance the clarity and detail of images.

Benefits: These nanoparticles improve the contrast in imaging, allowing for better visualization of cardiovascular structures and abnormalities.

Case Study: A study in Nature Nanotechnology demonstrated the use of gold nanoparticles in enhancing the contrast of CT scans, which improved the detection and diagnosis of cardiovascular diseases.

Gold's unique properties make it an invaluable resource in modern medical applications, particularly in the field of cardiovascular health. Its use in medical implants, targeted drug delivery systems, anti-inflammatory treatments, and advanced imaging techniques underscores its versatility and effectiveness. Ongoing research continues to explore new and innovative ways to harness gold's potential, promising further advancements in medical science.

Finger Placement for Wearing Gold to Balance the Circulatory System

In traditional practices, wearing gold on specific fingers is believed to influence various aspects of health, including the circulatory system. Here is a detailed look at which finger to wear gold on to help balance the circulatory system:

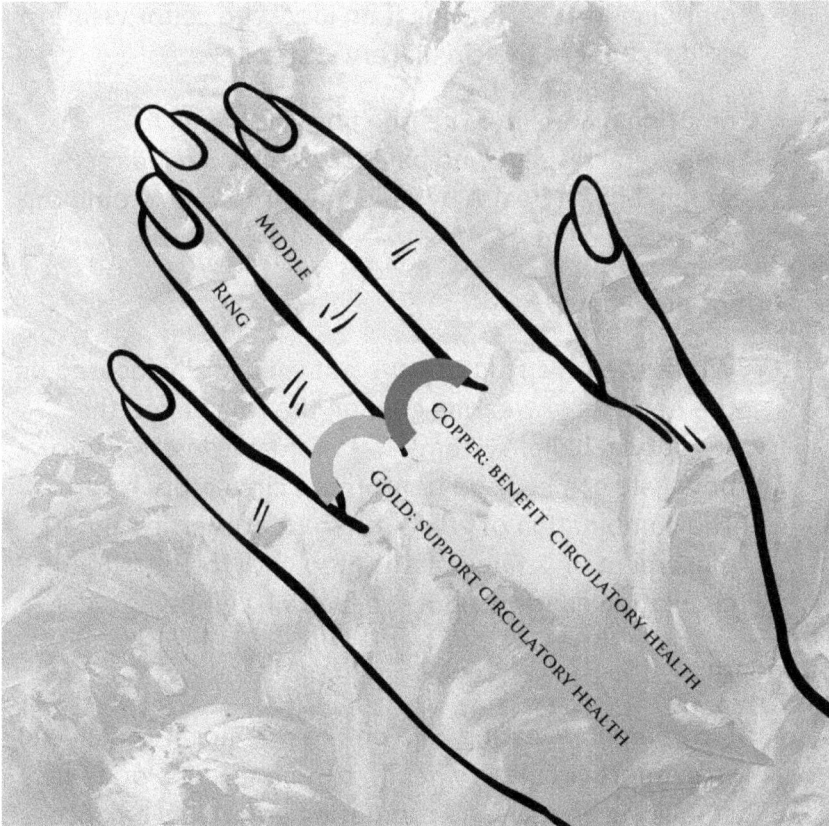

Ring Finger (Fourth Finger):

> Traditional Belief: In both Ayurvedic and TCM practices, the ring finger is associated with the Earth element, which is believed to ground and stabilize energy.

> Circulatory Health: Wearing gold on the ring finger is thought to enhance blood circulation and support the heart. The ring finger is also connected to the heart meridian in TCM, making it an ideal choice for wearing gold to benefit the circulatory system.

> Emotional Stability: The ring finger is linked to emotional stability and balance, which can indirectly support heart health by reducing stress and promoting a sense of calm.

Scientific Perspective:

> While scientific studies have not specifically focused on the benefits of wearing gold on the ring finger, the traditional belief system offers valuable insights into how gold can be used to promote circulatory health. The combination of gold's inherent properties and its placement on a finger associated with the heart and circulation can contribute to overall well-being.

Summary

> **Ring Finger:** Wearing gold on the ring finger is believed to support circulatory health by enhancing blood flow, stabilizing energy, and promoting emotional balance. This finger's connection to the heart meridian and its traditional association with emotional stability and balance align well with the beneficial properties of gold for the circulatory system.

Wearing gold on the ring finger is believed to support circulatory health by enhancing blood flow, stabilizing energy, and promoting emotional balance. This practice is rooted in traditional Ayurvedic and TCM beliefs, highlighting the holistic approach to using metals for health benefits. While modern science continues to explore the applications of gold in medicine, these traditional insights provide valuable guidance for those seeking to balance their circulatory system through the use of gold.

WESTERN PERSPECTIVE: SYMBOLISM OF THE RING FINGER
Western practice of wearing a gold ring on the ring finger (typically the fourth finger of the left hand) can differ in its cultural and symbolic significance. In many Western cultures, wearing a gold ring on the ring finger, especially the fourth finger of the left hand has a deep symbolic meaning:

Wedding and Engagement Rings: Traditionally, the left ring finger is reserved for wedding and engagement rings. This practice dates back to ancient Roman times when it was believed that the "vena amoris" (vein of love) ran directly from this finger to the heart.

Cultural and Religious Significance:

> In Western cultures, the gold ring symbolizes commitment, fidelity, and eternal love. It is a widely accepted practice in marriage ceremonies.

Why the Difference?

> Cultural and Historical Practices: The Western tradition of wearing rings on the ring finger is rooted in cultural and historical symbolism rather than health benefits. This tradition has been widely adopted and is less influenced by the energetic and health principles found in TCM and Ayurveda.

Symbolism vs. Energetics: In Western culture, the focus is more on the symbolism of the ring finger rather than the energetic influences on health. This contrasts with TCM and Ayurveda, where the placement of jewelry is more directly related to influencing health and energy balance.

Modern Adaptations: Today, people often blend practices from different cultures. While some may adhere strictly to TCM or Ayurvedic guidelines, others might follow Western traditions for personal or cultural reasons.

While TCM and Ayurveda provide guidelines on the placement of rings based on energetic and health principles, the Western practice of wearing a gold ring on the ring finger is largely symbolic and cultural. Both approaches have their unique significance, and individuals may choose their practices based on personal beliefs, cultural traditions, and health considerations.

Finger Placement for Wearing Copper to Support Circulatory Health

In traditional practices, wearing copper on specific fingers is believed to influence various aspects of health, particularly the circulatory system. Here is a detailed look at which finger to wear copper on to help balance and enhance circulatory health:

Middle Finger (Third Finger)

Traditional Belief: Ayurveda and TCM: The middle finger represents balance and core energy, which are associated with responsibility and structural stability. Wearing copper on this finger is believed to strengthen the body's core and improve the stability of its internal systems.

Circulatory Health: Strength and Stability: Wearing copper on the middle finger is thought to support the overall stability of the body's systems, including the circulatory system. By promoting structural balance, copper helps ensure that the heart and blood vessels function harmoniously.

Grounding Effect: Emotional and Physical Grounding: The middle finger's association with balance and strength aligns with copper's grounding properties, providing both emotional and physical support to the circulatory system.

Scientific Perspective

While scientific studies have not specifically focused on the benefits of wearing copper on particular fingers, traditional belief systems offer valuable insights into how copper can be used to support circulatory health. The combination of copper's inherent properties and its placement on fingers, which are associated with heart and energy flow, can contribute to overall well-being.

Summary

Middle Finger: Wearing copper on the middle finger is thought to benefit circulatory health by promoting balance, strength, and stability. This finger's association with core energy and structural integrity aligns with the supportive properties of copper.

These traditional practices highlight a unique perspective on using metals for health benefits. While modern science continues to explore the applications of copper in medicine, these insights provide valuable guidance for those seeking to balance their circulatory system through the use of copper.

Chapter 7:
The Respiratory System

Overview of the Respiratory System

The respiratory system is essential for breathing and the exchange of gases between the body and the environment. It is responsible for bringing oxygen into the body and expelling carbon dioxide, a waste product of metabolism. The respiratory system includes the nose, throat, larynx (voice box), trachea (windpipe), bronchi, and lungs. The primary functions of the respiratory system are:

- Gas Exchange: Facilitating the exchange of oxygen and carbon dioxide between the air and the bloodstream.
- Air Filtration: Filtering and trapping dust, microbes, and other particulates from the air we breathe.
- Regulation of pH: Helping maintain the acid-base balance of the blood by regulating the levels of carbon dioxide.
- Voice Production: Producing sounds for speech by passing air over the vocal cords in the larynx.
- Olfaction: Enabling the sense of smell through the nasal passages.

METAL TO BALANCE THE RESPIRATORY SYSTEM
SILVER: THE LUNGS AND AIRWAYS

BENEFITS OF SILVER FOR THE RESPIRATORY SYSTEM

Antimicrobial Action: When used in respiratory treatments, silver can help eliminate harmful microbes in the airways. This is particularly beneficial in preventing and treating respiratory infections like bronchitis, pneumonia, and the common cold.

Reducing Inflammation: Inhaling silver particles or using silver-based nasal sprays can reduce inflammation in the respiratory tract, making breathing easier and relieving symptoms of conditions like asthma and chronic obstructive pulmonary disease (COPD).

Improving Lung Health: Silver can help maintain the overall health of the lungs by preventing infections and reducing inflammation. This is particularly useful for people with weakened immune systems or chronic respiratory conditions.

SAFETY AND CONSIDERATIONS

While silver has many benefits, it is important to use it responsibly:

Proper Dosage: Overuse of silver, especially colloidal silver, can lead to a condition called argyria, where the skin turns a bluish-gray color. It's crucial to follow recommended dosages.

Consult a Healthcare Provider: Before using silver-based products, especially for respiratory conditions, consult a healthcare provider to ensure it's appropriate for your specific situation.

Traditional Uses of Silver for Respiratory Health

Silver has been used for centuries in various cultures for its medicinal properties, particularly in promoting respiratory health. Here are some traditional uses of silver for respiratory health:

ANTIMICROBIAL PROPERTIES
Colloidal Silver:

> Colloidal silver is a suspension of fine silver particles in water. It has been used traditionally as an antimicrobial agent to treat respiratory infections. People have used it to gargle for sore throats, as a nasal spray for sinus infections, and orally to boost the immune system.

Silver Vessels:

> Drinking water from silver vessels has been a common practice in some cultures, believed to purify the water and provide antimicrobial benefits that can aid in preventing respiratory infections.

ANTI-INFLAMMATORY EFFECTS
Inhalation Therapy:

> Inhaling steam infused with colloidal silver has been used to reduce inflammation in the respiratory tract, helping to ease symptoms of conditions like bronchitis and asthma.

Topical Applications:

> Silver-based ointments have been applied to the chest to reduce inflammation and congestion, often combined with other herbal remedies.

PREVENTIVE MEASURES
Silverware:

> Historically, the use of silverware for eating and drinking was thought to provide continuous low-level exposure to silver, which helped prevent respiratory and other infections.

Air Purification:

> In some cultures, placing silver items in water fountains or air purification systems was believed to help disinfect the air, thereby reducing the spread of airborne pathogens and improving respiratory health.

WOUND HEALING AND RECOVERY
Silver Dressings:

> Silver-infused dressings have been used to treat wounds and prevent infections. For respiratory health, these dressings might be applied to surgical wounds or injuries in the chest area to prevent infections that could complicate breathing.

Modern Applications and Case Studies

MODERN ADAPTATIONS OF TRADITIONAL USES
Nebulizers and Inhalers:

> Modern adaptations include nebulizers and inhalers that can deliver colloidal silver directly to the lungs, offering a contemporary approach to traditional inhalation therapies.

Silver-Infused Masks:

> In response to recent health crises, silver-infused masks have been developed to provide antimicrobial protection, drawing from the traditional use of silver's antimicrobial properties to protect respiratory health.

Colloidal Silver Supplements:

> Colloidal silver is available in liquid form and is used as a dietary supplement. It is often marketed for its purported benefits in boosting the immune system and treating respiratory infections.

Silver-Infused Medical Devices:

> Many medical devices, such as catheters, wound dressings, and breathing tubes, are infused with silver to prevent infections. The antimicrobial properties of silver help reduce the risk of hospital-acquired infections.

Topical Silver Products:

> Silver sulfadiazine cream is widely used to treat burns and prevent wound infections. It promotes healing and reduces the risk of bacterial contamination.

Silver-Embedded Textiles:

> Clothing and textiles embedded with silver fibers are used in healthcare settings to reduce microbial growth on fabrics, thus helping to prevent the spread of infections.

Silver-Infused Air Purifiers and Filters:

> Air purifiers and filters with silver nanoparticles are used to kill bacteria and viruses in the air, improving indoor air quality and reducing the risk of respiratory infections.

Silver Nanoparticles in Coatings:

> Silver nanoparticles are used in coatings for various surfaces, including medical instruments, to provide long-lasting antimicrobial protection.

CASE STUDIES

Case Study: Silver-Coated Endotracheal Tubes:

> Background: Ventilator-associated pneumonia (VAP) is a significant risk for patients on mechanical ventilation. Silver-coated endotracheal tubes have been developed to mitigate this risk.

> Study: A study published in the journal Chest examined the effectiveness of silver-coated endotracheal tubes in preventing VAP.

> Results: The study found a significant reduction in the incidence of VAP among patients using silver-coated tubes compared to those using standard tubes. The silver coating helped reduce bacterial colonization on the tubes, thereby lowering infection rates.

Case Study: Silver-Impregnated Wound Dressings:

> Background: Chronic wounds, such as diabetic ulcers and pressure sores, are prone to infections and require effective management to promote healing.

> Study: Research published in the Journal of Wound Care evaluated the effectiveness of silver-impregnated wound dressings in managing chronic wounds.

> Results: Patients treated with silver-impregnated dressings showed faster healing times and lower infection rates compared to those treated with non-silver dressings. The antimicrobial properties of silver helped control bacterial growth in the wound area.

Case Study: Silver Nanoparticles in Air Filters:

> Background: Indoor air quality is crucial for preventing respiratory infections, especially in healthcare settings.

> Study: A study conducted by researchers at the University of Southampton investigated the efficacy of air filters coated with silver nanoparticles in reducing airborne pathogens.

> Results: The silver nanoparticle-coated filters demonstrated a significant reduction in bacterial and viral counts in the air. This application is particularly beneficial in hospital environments to reduce the spread of infections.

Case Study: Silver Nanoparticles in Antimicrobial Coatings:

> Background: Medical instruments and surfaces are common sources of hospital-acquired infections.

> Study: A study published in the International Journal of Nanomedicine explored the use of silver nanoparticles in antimicrobial coatings for medical instruments.

> Results: Instruments coated with silver nanoparticles showed a marked reduction in microbial contamination compared to uncoated instruments. The silver coatings provided long-lasting antimicrobial effects, making them suitable for use in high-touch areas of healthcare facilities.

Modern applications of silver leverage its powerful antimicrobial and anti-inflammatory properties to improve health outcomes and prevent infections. From silver-coated medical devices and wound dressings to air purifiers and antimicrobial coatings, silver plays a crucial role in contemporary healthcare. These applications are supported by numerous case studies demonstrating their effectiveness in reducing infection rates and promoting healing, validating the continued relevance of silver in modern medicine.

Finger Placement for Wearing Silver to Support Respiratory Health

In traditional practices, wearing silver on specific fingers is believed to influence various aspects of health, including the respiratory system. Here is a detailed look at which finger to wear silver on to help support respiratory health:

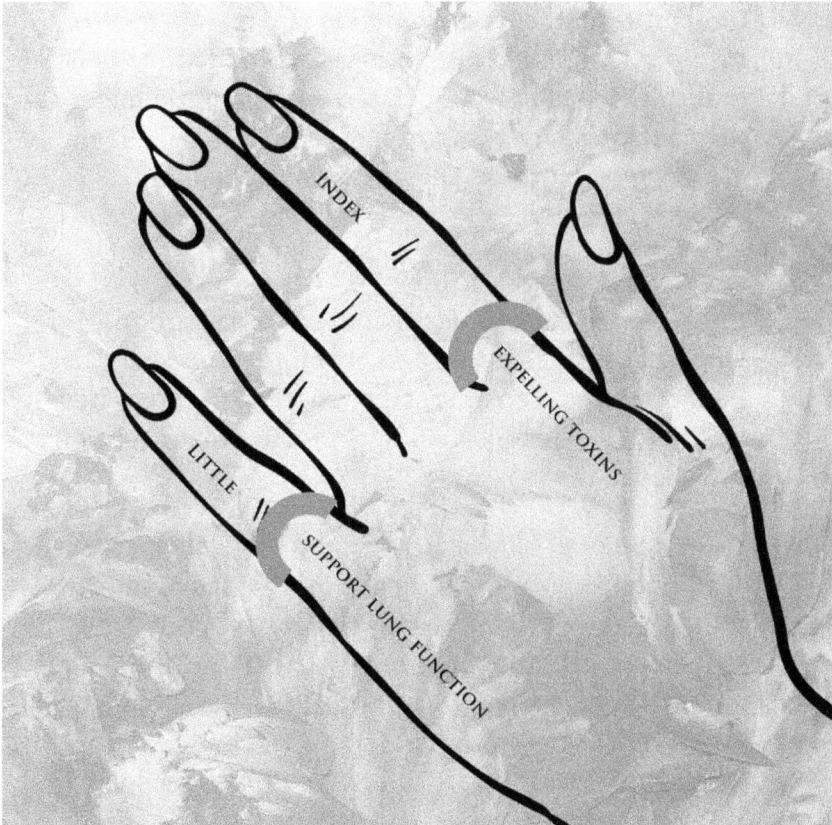

LITTLE FINGER (FIFTH FINGER):
Traditional Belief: In both Ayurvedic and Traditional Chinese Medicine (TCM) practices, the little finger is associated with the Water element. This element is connected to the health of the kidneys and lungs. In TCM, the little finger is also linked to the heart and small intestine meridians, which are believed to indirectly influence respiratory health.

> Respiratory Health: Wearing silver on the little finger is thought to support lung function and enhance respiratory health. This practice is rooted in the belief that the energy flow associated with the little finger can help balance and strengthen the lungs, making it an ideal choice for those seeking to improve their respiratory system.

> Calm and Relaxation: The little finger is also linked to the ability to communicate and express emotions, which can reduce stress and promote a sense of calm. Reduced stress can indirectly benefit respiratory health by improving overall well-being and reducing tension in the chest and lungs.

INDEX FINGER (SECOND FINGER):
> Traditional Belief: The index finger is associated with the Air element in Ayurveda, which governs the movement and flow of energy in the body. In TCM, the index finger is linked to the large intestine meridian, which is considered to have an impact on the respiratory system, particularly in terms of expelling toxins and waste.

> Respiratory Health: Wearing silver on the index finger can help enhance respiratory health by supporting the expulsion of toxins and improving overall airflow within

the body. This can be beneficial for clearing the respiratory pathways and promoting easier breathing.

Energy Flow: The index finger is related to personal power and assertiveness. By balancing energy flow, wearing silver on this finger can help maintain a strong and resilient respiratory system.

Scientific Perspective:

While there are no specific scientific studies focused on the benefits of wearing silver on particular fingers, traditional belief systems provide valuable insights into how silver can be used to support respiratory health. The combination of silver's antimicrobial properties and its placement on fingers, which are associated with lung health and energy flow, can contribute to overall well-being.

Summary:

Little Finger: (TCM/Ayurvedic): Wearing silver on the little finger is believed to support lung function, promote respiratory health, and enhance calm and relaxation.

Index Finger: Wearing silver on the index finger is thought to aid in expelling toxins, improving airflow, and maintaining a strong respiratory system.

These practices are rooted in traditional Ayurvedic and TCM beliefs, highlighting a holistic approach to using metals for health benefits. While modern science continues to explore the applications of silver in medicine, these traditional insights offer valuable guidance for those seeking to support their respiratory system through the use of silver.

Chapter 8:
The Digestive System

Overview of the Digestive System

The digestive system is essential for breaking down food, absorbing nutrients, and eliminating waste from the body. It consists of several organs that work together to convert food into energy and essential nutrients that the body needs to function properly. The digestive system includes the mouth, esophagus, stomach, small intestine, large intestine, liver, pancreas, and gallbladder. The primary functions of the digestive system are:

- o Digestion: Breaking down food into smaller molecules that can be absorbed.
- o Absorption: Absorbing nutrients and water into the bloodstream for use by the body.
- o Elimination: Removing waste products and undigested food from the body.

METAL TO BALANCE THE DIGESTIVE SYSTEM
COPPER: THE STOMACH AND LIVER

BENEFITS OF COPPER FOR DIGESTION
Copper

> Antimicrobial Properties: Copper has natural antimicrobial properties, which help kill harmful bacteria and pathogens that can disrupt the digestive system.

> Enzyme Production: Copper aids in the production of digestive enzymes, which are essential for breaking down food and absorbing nutrients effectively.

> Improves Gut Health: Copper supports the maintenance of a healthy gut lining, reducing the risk of inflammation and ulcers.

> Helps with Peristalsis: Copper can stimulate peristalsis, the wave-like muscle contractions that move food through the digestive tract, ensuring smooth digestion and preventing constipation.

BENEFITS OF STAINLESS STEEL FOR DIGESTION
Stainless Steel

> Antimicrobial Properties: Inhibition of Pathogens: Stainless steel surfaces naturally inhibit the growth of bacteria, viruses, and fungi, which can help maintain a healthier environment and reduce the risk of digestive infections.

> Food Safety: Using stainless steel in kitchen environments ensures that surfaces remain free from

harmful microbes, protecting the digestive system from foodborne illnesses.

SAFETY AND CONSIDERATIONS FOR COPPER IN DIGESTION
Copper

Copper Toxicity: Excessive intake of copper can lead to copper toxicity, which can cause symptoms such as nausea, vomiting, abdominal pain, and diarrhea. It's important to ensure that copper is consumed in moderation.

Proper Usage: Use copper utensils and cookware appropriately to avoid excessive copper intake. Cooking highly acidic foods in copper pots can cause more copper to leach into the food.

Maintenance: Copper utensils should be properly maintained and cleaned. Oxidation and patina on copper surfaces can harbor bacteria if not cleaned regularly.

Medical Conditions: Individuals with certain medical conditions, such as Wilson's disease, should avoid using copper utensils and cookware, as they have difficulty regulating copper levels in the body.

SAFETY AND CONSIDERATIONS FOR STAINLESS STEEL IN DIGESTION
Stainless Steel

Potential Allergies: Nickel Sensitivity: Some individuals may have a sensitivity or allergy to nickel, which is often present in stainless steel alloys. Symptoms can include skin irritation, rashes, or gastrointestinal discomfort. If you have a known nickel allergy, look for stainless steel labeled as "nickel-free" or consider alternative materials.

Traditional Uses of Copper in Digestion

Copper has been utilized for centuries in various cultures for its beneficial effects on health, particularly in supporting the digestive system. Here are some traditional uses of copper in digestion:

ANTIMICROBIAL PROPERTIES
Copper Vessels and Utensils:

In Ayurveda, it is common to drink water stored in copper vessels. This practice is believed to harness copper's antimicrobial properties, killing harmful bacteria and purifying the water. Drinking copper-infused water, known as "tamra jal," can help maintain gut health by reducing the risk of gastrointestinal infections.

Copper Cookware:

Cooking with copper pots and pans is another traditional practice. The antimicrobial action of copper can help reduce the bacterial load in food, thereby supporting digestive health. Copper cookware also ensures even heat distribution, which can help in the proper cooking of food and aid in digestion.

ANTI-INFLAMMATORY EFFECTS
Alleviating Inflammation:

Traditional medicine systems like Ayurveda suggest that copper can help reduce inflammation in the stomach and intestines. This anti-inflammatory effect can alleviate symptoms of digestive disorders such as gastritis and irritable bowel syndrome (IBS).

ENZYMATIC SUPPORT
Supporting Digestive Enzymes:

Copper is an essential co-factor for many enzymes involved in the digestive process. Traditional practices emphasize the importance of maintaining adequate copper levels to support these enzymatic activities, which help in the breakdown and absorption of nutrients.

DETOXIFICATION
Liver Health:

Copper plays a crucial role in the detoxification processes of the liver. In traditional practices, maintaining proper copper levels is believed to support liver function, aiding in the detoxification of harmful substances and promoting overall digestive health.

HEALING PROPERTIES
Wound Healing in the Digestive Tract:

Copper has been traditionally used to promote healing. Its properties are thought to assist in the repair of the lining of the digestive tract, helping to heal ulcers and other gastrointestinal lesions.

BALANCING DOSHAS
Tridoshic Balance:

In Ayurveda, copper is considered beneficial for balancing the three doshas (Vata, Pitta, and Kapha). Drinking water from copper vessels is believed to help maintain this balance, contributing to overall digestive harmony and well-being.

Copper's traditional uses in supporting digestion highlight its significant role in maintaining gastrointestinal health. From antimicrobial properties and enzyme support to anti-inflammatory effects and detoxification, copper has been a valuable element in traditional health practices.

Modern Applications and Case

Copper continues to be an essential element in modern health practices, particularly in supporting the digestive system. Here are some of the key modern applications of copper and relevant case studies:

MODERN APPLICATIONS
Copper-Infused Water Bottles and Vessels:

> Modern versions of traditional copper vessels, such as copper-infused water bottles, have become popular. These bottles are designed to purify water and provide the antimicrobial benefits of copper, supporting overall digestive health. Users are advised to fill the bottle with water and let it sit overnight to allow the copper ions to infuse the water.

Copper Supplements:

> Copper supplements are available in various forms, such as capsules, tablets, and liquid drops. These supplements can help ensure adequate copper intake, especially for individuals with dietary deficiencies. They are often recommended under the guidance of healthcare providers to avoid toxicity.

Copper-Infused Textiles and Surfaces:

> Copper-infused textiles and surfaces are used in healthcare settings to reduce microbial contamination. For example, copper-infused hospital bedsheets and surfaces can help prevent the spread of infections, indirectly supporting the digestive health of patients by reducing the risk of hospital-acquired infections.

Copper-Enhanced Foods:

> Some food products are fortified with copper to enhance their nutritional value. These include certain cereals, health bars, and dietary supplements. These products are designed to help meet daily copper requirements, supporting enzymatic functions and overall digestive health.

Safety and Considerations

> While traditional uses of copper offer various benefits for digestion, it is important to use copper responsibly:

> Proper Dosage: Excessive copper intake can lead to toxicity. It is crucial to follow recommended dietary allowances and consult a healthcare provider if considering supplements.

> Balanced Diet: Ensure a balanced diet that includes other essential minerals and nutrients to avoid imbalances and potential health issues.

CASE STUDIES

Case Study: Copper Water Bottles and Gastrointestinal Health:

> Background: A study was conducted to evaluate the impact of drinking water from copper vessels on gastrointestinal health.

Method: Participants were provided with copper water bottles and instructed to drink water stored in these bottles overnight for a period of 30 days.

Results: The study observed a reduction in gastrointestinal infections and improvements in digestion among participants. The antimicrobial properties of copper were effective in reducing harmful bacteria in the water, contributing to better digestive health.

Case Study: Copper Supplements and Liver Function:

Background: Research investigating the effects of copper supplementation on liver function in individuals with copper deficiency.

Method: Copper-deficient individuals were given copper supplements for a period of 8 weeks.

Results: The study found significant improvements in liver enzyme levels and overall liver function. The supplements helped restore copper levels, supporting the liver's role in detoxification and metabolism, which are crucial for digestive health.

Case Study: Copper-Infused Surfaces in Healthcare:

Background: An investigation into the effectiveness of copper-infused surfaces in reducing hospital-acquired infections.

Method: Copper-infused surfaces were installed in a hospital ward, and infection rates were monitored over six months.

Results: The incidence of hospital-acquired infections decreased by 58% in the ward with copper-infused surfaces compared to a control ward. This reduction in infections indirectly supported the digestive health of patients by lowering the risk of gastrointestinal pathogens.

Case Study: Copper in Food Fortification:

Background: A study on the impact of copper-fortified foods on dietary copper intake and digestive health.

Method: Participants consumed copper-fortified cereals and health bars for 12 weeks.

Results: The study showed an increase in dietary copper intake and improvements in digestive enzyme activity. Participants reported better digestion and fewer digestive issues, highlighting the benefits of copper fortification in food products.

Modern applications of copper continue to build on traditional knowledge, leveraging its antimicrobial, enzymatic, and healing properties to support digestive health. From copper-infused water bottles and supplements to copper-enhanced foods and surfaces, these applications are supported by scientific research and case studies demonstrating their effectiveness. By integrating these modern practices, individuals can benefit from the digestive health-supporting properties of copper, ensuring a holistic approach to wellness that blends tradition with contemporary science.

Finger Placement for Wearing Copper to Support Digestive Health

In traditional practices, wearing copper on specific fingers is believed to influence various aspects of health, including the digestive system. Here is a detailed look at which finger to wear copper on to help support digestive health:

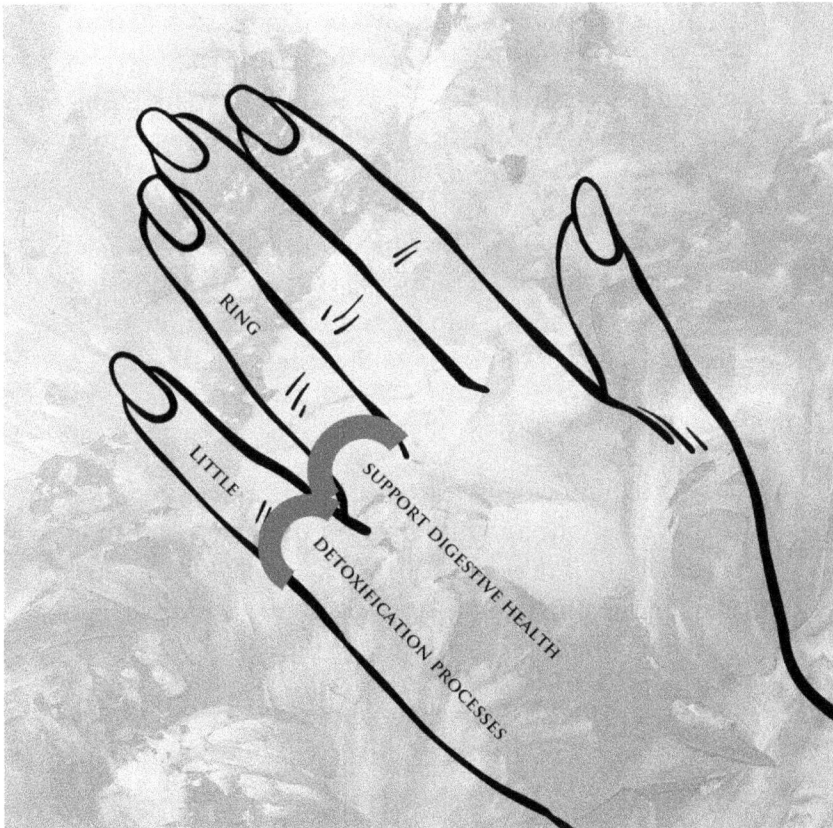

Ring Finger (Fourth Finger):

> Traditional Belief: In both Ayurvedic and Traditional Chinese Medicine (TCM) practices, the ring finger is associated with the Earth element. The Earth element is linked to stability, grounding, and nourishment, all of which are crucial for a healthy digestive system.

> Digestive Health: Wearing copper on the ring finger is thought to enhance digestive processes and support the functions of the stomach and liver. The Earth element's grounding energy is believed to help balance the digestive system, improving nutrient absorption and waste elimination.

> Emotional Stability: The ring finger is also connected to emotional stability. Emotional balance can indirectly benefit digestive health by reducing stress, which is a common factor in digestive disorders.

Little Finger (Fifth Finger):

> Traditional Belief: The little finger is associated with the Water element in Ayurveda and the heart and small intestine meridians in TCM. This finger is believed to influence fluid balance and metabolic processes, both of which are important for digestion.

> Digestive Health: Wearing copper on the little finger can support liver function and the body's detoxification processes. It is thought to aid in the elimination of toxins and improve the efficiency of the digestive system, particularly in the processing of fats.

> Communication and Stress Relief: The little finger is also linked to communication and stress relief. Reducing stress through improved emotional expression can

positively impact digestive health by minimizing the effects of stress on the gastrointestinal tract.

Scientific Perspective

While there are no specific scientific studies focused on the benefits of wearing copper on particular fingers, traditional belief systems provide valuable insights into how copper can be used to support digestive health. The combination of copper's antimicrobial and enzymatic properties, along with its placement on fingers associated with digestive balance, can contribute to overall well-being.

Summary

Ring Finger: Wearing copper on the ring finger is believed to support digestive health by enhancing nutrient absorption, waste elimination, and emotional stability. This practice is rooted in the connection between the Earth element and the digestive system.

Little Finger: Wearing copper on the little finger is thought to aid liver function, detoxification processes, and stress relief, all of which are beneficial for maintaining a healthy digestive system.

These practices are rooted in traditional Ayurvedic and TCM beliefs, highlighting a holistic approach to using metals for health benefits. While modern science continues to explore the applications of copper in medicine, these traditional insights offer valuable guidance for those seeking to support their digestive system through the use of copper.

Finger Placement for Wearing Stainless Steel to Support Digestive Health

In traditional and modern holistic practices, wearing metals on specific fingers is believed to influence various aspects of health, including digestive health. Stainless steel, known for its durability, non-reactivity, and hygienic properties, can be beneficial when worn as a ring on specific fingers to support the digestive system. Here is a detailed look at which finger to wear stainless steel on to help support digestive health:

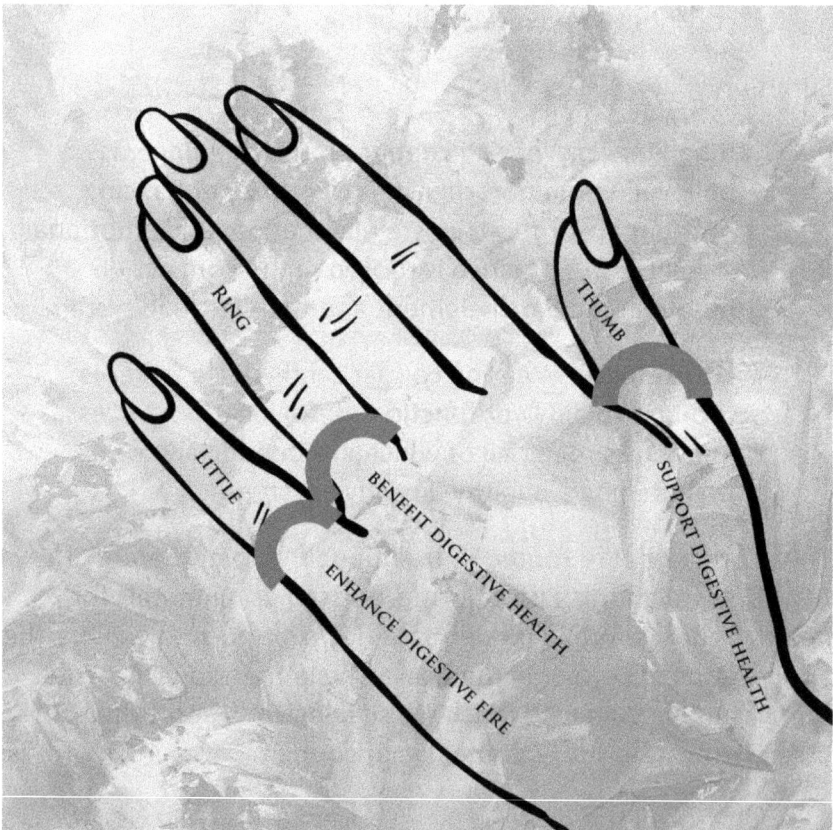

Ring Finger (Fourth Finger)

Traditional Belief: The ring finger is associated with the Earth element in both Ayurvedic and Traditional Chinese Medicine (TCM). This element is linked to stability, grounding, and the digestive system.

Digestive Health: Wearing stainless steel on the ring finger is believed to enhance digestion, support nutrient absorption, and promote overall gastrointestinal health. The ring finger's connection to the Earth element makes it an ideal choice for addressing issues related to the stomach and intestines.

Emotional Stability: The ring finger is also linked to emotional stability, which can indirectly support digestive health by reducing stress and promoting a sense of calm.

Middle Finger (Third Finger)

Traditional Belief: The middle finger represents balance and the body's core energy. It is associated with responsibility and structure, essential for maintaining the body's internal systems, including the digestive system.

Digestive Health: Wearing stainless steel on the middle finger is thought to support the overall balance and stability of the body's systems. This can indirectly benefit the digestive system by ensuring that the stomach and intestines function harmoniously within the body's regulatory processes.

Strength and Stability: The middle finger's symbolism of strength and stability can help reinforce the body's ability to manage digestive health efficiently.

Thumb (First Finger)

> Traditional Belief: The thumb is associated with the element of Fire in TCM, which is linked to the stomach and digestive fire (Agni) in Ayurveda. This element governs metabolism and the digestive process.

> Digestive Health: Wearing stainless steel on the thumb is believed to enhance digestive fire, improving metabolism and the breakdown of food. The thumb's connection to the Fire element makes it a suitable choice for addressing sluggish digestion and boosting digestive efficiency.

> Metabolic Support: The thumb's association with digestive fire aligns with its role in supporting metabolic health and energy production.

Scientific Perspective

While specific scientific studies focused on the benefits of wearing stainless steel on particular fingers are limited, traditional belief systems provide valuable insights into how stainless steel can be used to support digestive health. The combination of stainless steel's hygienic and non-reactive properties, along with its placement on fingers associated with digestive health, can contribute to overall well-being.

Summary

Ring Finger: Wearing stainless steel on the ring finger is believed to support digestive health by enhancing digestion, nutrient absorption, and promoting gastrointestinal stability.

Middle Finger: Wearing stainless steel on the middle finger is thought to benefit digestive health by promoting balance, strength, and stability within the body's regulatory processes.

Thumb: Wearing stainless steel on the thumb is believed to enhance digestive fire, supporting metabolism and the efficient breakdown of food.

These practices are rooted in traditional beliefs and holistic approaches, highlighting a unique perspective on using metals for health benefits. While modern science continues to explore the applications of stainless steel in medicine, these traditional insights offer valuable guidance for those seeking to support their digestive health through the use of metal jewelry.

Chapter 9:
The Nervous System

Overview of the Nervous System

The nervous system is essential for coordinating and controlling the activities of the body. It is responsible for processing sensory information, initiating responses, and regulating bodily functions. The nervous system includes the brain, spinal cord, and a network of nerves that extend throughout the body. The primary functions of the nervous system are:

- Control and Coordination: Regulating bodily functions and responses to internal and external stimuli.
- Sensory Input: Receiving and processing sensory information from the environment.
- Motor Output: Initiating and controlling movement.
- Cognitive Functions: Supporting thought processes, memory, learning, and emotions.

Metal To Balance The Nervous System
Platinum: The Brain And Nerves

Benefits Of Platinum For The Nervous System
Neuroprotective Effects:

> Research suggests that platinum compounds may have neuroprotective effects, helping to protect brain cells from damage and degeneration. This could be beneficial in treating neurodegenerative diseases such as Alzheimer's and Parkinson's.

Medical Implants:

> Platinum is used in various medical implants, such as deep brain stimulators and spinal cord stimulators. These devices help manage neurological conditions by delivering electrical impulses to specific areas of the brain or spinal cord.

Cancer Treatment:

> Platinum-based drugs, such as cisplatin, are used in chemotherapy to treat various cancers, including brain tumors. These drugs help destroy cancer cells and prevent their spread.

Electrodes and Sensors:

> Platinum electrodes and sensors are used in medical devices to monitor and stimulate neural activity. These devices are critical in the research and treatment of neurological disorders.

SAFETY AND CONSIDERATIONS

While platinum offers numerous benefits, it is important to use it responsibly:

> Medical Supervision: Platinum-based treatments and implants should be administered and monitored by qualified healthcare professionals.

> Potential Side Effects: Platinum-based drugs can have side effects, including nephrotoxicity (kidney damage) and neurotoxicity (nerve damage). Regular monitoring and dosage adjustments are essential.

Traditional Uses of Platinum for Mental Clarity

Platinum, a precious and rare metal, has been revered in various cultures for its potential benefits to mental clarity and overall cognitive function. Although its traditional uses are less well-documented compared to other metals like gold and silver, platinum has held a place in the realms of alchemy, ancient medicine, and holistic practices. Here are some traditional uses of platinum for enhancing mental clarity:

ALCHEMY AND SYMBOLISM

Alchemy:

> In ancient alchemy, platinum was considered a metal of transformation and purity. Alchemists believed that platinum possessed unique energies that could enhance mental clarity and spiritual awareness. It was often associated with achieving higher states of consciousness and was used in various alchemical preparations aimed at refining the mind and spirit.

Symbolic Significance:

> Platinum has been a symbol of excellence, durability, and clarity. Its rarity and purity were thought to mirror the qualities of a clear and focused mind. Wearing or carrying platinum was believed to align one's mental energies with these attributes, promoting sharper thinking and greater mental resilience.

AYURVEDA AND TRADITIONAL MEDICINE
Ayurvedic Medicine:

> Although not as commonly referenced as other metals, some Ayurvedic traditions have included platinum in their repertoire of beneficial metals. It was sometimes used in combination with other herbs and minerals in rasayanas (rejuvenative tonics), believed to enhance cognitive functions and mental clarity.

Mental Balance and Focus:

> In traditional medicine systems, metals like platinum were sometimes incorporated into amulets and talismans worn to balance mental energies. The inherent stability and strength of platinum were thought to provide mental grounding and focus, helping individuals maintain clarity in thought and action.

HOLISTIC AND METAPHYSICAL PRACTICES
Crystal and Metal Healing:

> In holistic healing practices, platinum is considered to have a high vibrational frequency that can influence the mind. It is used in energy healing and meditation practices to clear mental fog, enhance concentration, and promote a state of mental calm and clarity. Practitioners might use platinum-infused tools or

jewelry during meditation to harness its purported mental benefits.

Meditative Practices:

Platinum's reflective properties are believed to aid in meditative practices. It is thought to help reflect one's inner thoughts and bring subconscious ideas to the forefront, thereby aiding in mental clarity and self-awareness.

Modern Applications and Case Studies

Platinum continues to be a subject of interest in modern medical and technological fields due to its unique properties. Although direct scientific evidence linking platinum to mental clarity is limited, its applications in medical treatments and devices suggest potential cognitive benefits. Here, we explore the modern applications and relevant case studies of platinum in the context of brain and nerve health.

MODERN APPLICATIONS
Platinum-Based Medications:

Neuroprotective Agents: Research is ongoing into the use of platinum compounds as neuroprotective agents. These compounds are being studied for their potential to protect brain cells from damage and degeneration, which could indirectly support cognitive functions and mental clarity.

Chemotherapy Drugs: Platinum-based drugs like cisplatin, carboplatin, and oxaliplatin are commonly used in chemotherapy to treat various cancers, including brain tumors. While primarily targeting cancer cells, these drugs have highlighted the systemic effects platinum can have on the body and brain.

Medical Implants and Devices:

> Deep Brain Stimulation (DBS): Platinum electrodes are used in DBS devices, which deliver electrical impulses to specific brain areas to treat neurological conditions like Parkinson's disease, essential tremor, and epilepsy. Patients often report improvements in cognitive function and mental clarity as a secondary benefit of symptom relief.

> Neural Prosthetics: Platinum is used in neural prosthetics designed to restore lost sensory or motor functions. These devices can help improve the quality of life for individuals with nerve damage, potentially enhancing mental clarity through better neurological function.

Platinum Nanoparticles:

> Drug Delivery Systems: Platinum nanoparticles are being researched for use in targeted drug delivery systems. These systems aim to deliver medications directly to specific brain regions, potentially enhancing the efficacy of treatments for neurological disorders and preserving cognitive functions.

> Diagnostic Tools: Platinum nanoparticles are also used in advanced diagnostic tools, improving the detection and monitoring of neurological diseases. Early diagnosis and monitoring can lead to better management of these conditions, indirectly supporting mental clarity.

Case Studies

Case Study: Platinum-Based Chemotherapy and Cognitive Function:

> Background: Research has investigated the cognitive side effects of platinum-based chemotherapy drugs like cisplatin.

> Method: Patients undergoing chemotherapy for brain tumors were monitored for cognitive changes.

> Results: While cisplatin effectively reduced tumor size, some patients experienced cognitive side effects, including "chemo brain" (cognitive impairment associated with chemotherapy). This highlights the complex relationship between platinum compounds and cognitive function, suggesting a need for further research into minimizing side effects while maximizing therapeutic benefits.

Case Study: Deep Brain Stimulation (DBS) for Parkinson's Disease:

> Background: DBS involves the implantation of platinum electrodes in the brain to alleviate symptoms of Parkinson's disease.

> Method: Patients with advanced Parkinson's disease received DBS treatment, and their cognitive and motor functions were evaluated.

> Results: Many patients reported significant improvements in motor function and a reduction in tremors and rigidity. Additionally, some patients experienced enhanced cognitive function and mental

clarity, likely due to improved overall neurological function and reduced disease symptoms.

Case Study: Platinum Nanoparticles in Drug Delivery:

Background: Research focused on using platinum nanoparticles to enhance the delivery of neuroprotective drugs to the brain.

Method: Animal models with induced neurodegenerative conditions were treated with drugs delivered via platinum nanoparticles.

Results: The studies showed improved drug efficacy, with enhanced protection of brain cells and better preservation of cognitive functions. This indicates that platinum nanoparticles can potentially support mental clarity by optimizing drug delivery to the brain.

Modern applications of platinum in medical treatments and devices offer promising avenues for supporting brain and nerve health, which can indirectly enhance mental clarity. While traditional beliefs about platinum's benefits for mental clarity are intriguing, modern scientific research is focusing on practical applications such as platinum-based medications, medical implants, and nanoparticles. These applications are supported by ongoing research and case studies, highlighting the potential cognitive benefits of platinum in treating neurological disorders and enhancing overall brain function. As research progresses, platinum's role in supporting mental clarity may become more clearly defined, blending traditional insights with contemporary scientific advancements.

Finger Placement for Wearing Platinum to Support Mental Clarity

In traditional and modern holistic practices, wearing platinum on specific fingers is believed to influence various aspects of health, including mental clarity and cognitive function. Here is a detailed look at which finger to wear platinum on to help support mental clarity:

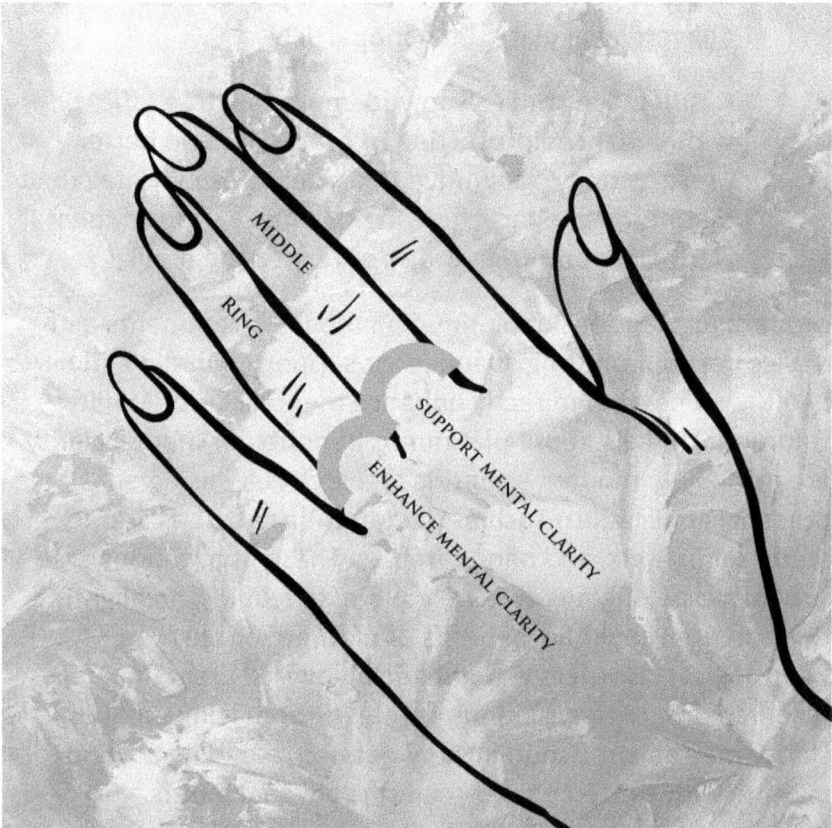

Ring Finger (Fourth Finger):

> Traditional Belief: In many cultures, the ring finger is associated with the Earth element, which represents grounding and stability. This grounding effect can help stabilize mental energies and enhance cognitive function.

> Mental Clarity: Wearing platinum on the ring finger is thought to promote mental clarity by providing a stabilizing influence. The grounding energy associated with this finger can help reduce mental stress and improve focus and concentration.

> Emotional Stability: The ring finger is also linked to emotional balance. Emotional stability can indirectly support mental clarity by reducing anxiety and promoting a calm and focused mind.

Middle Finger (Third Finger):

> Traditional Belief: The middle finger is associated with the balance and the body's core energies. It is linked to the Saturn planet, which represents discipline, responsibility, and clarity of thought.

> Mental Clarity: Wearing platinum on the middle finger is believed to enhance mental clarity by promoting a sense of balance and discipline. This can help improve decision-making, problem-solving abilities, and overall cognitive function.

> Strength and Stability: The middle finger is the strongest finger and is thought to symbolize strength and stability. Wearing platinum on this finger can help harness these qualities to support a clear and focused mind.

Scientific Perspective

> While there are no specific scientific studies focused on the benefits of wearing platinum on particular fingers, traditional belief systems provide valuable insights into how platinum can be used to support mental clarity. The combination of platinum's symbolic properties and its placement on fingers, which are associated with stability and balance, can contribute to overall mental well-being.

Summary

> **Ring Finger:** Wearing platinum on the ring finger is believed to support mental clarity by providing grounding and emotional stability. This practice is rooted in the connection between the Earth element and cognitive function.

> **Middle Finger**: Wearing platinum on the middle finger is thought to enhance mental clarity by promoting balance, discipline, and stability. This finger is associated with strength and core energies, making it an ideal choice for supporting cognitive function.

These practices are rooted in traditional beliefs and holistic approaches, highlighting a unique perspective on using metals for mental benefits. While modern science continues to explore the applications of platinum in medicine, these traditional insights offer valuable guidance for those seeking to support their mental clarity through the use of platinum.

Chapter 10:
The Skeletal System

Overview of the Skeletal System

The skeletal system is essential for providing structure, support, and protection to the human body. It enables movement, produces blood cells, and stores essential minerals. The skeletal system includes bones, joints, cartilage, ligaments, and tendons. The primary functions of the skeletal system are:

- o **Support and Structure**: Providing a rigid framework that supports the body and maintains its shape.
- o **Movement**: Facilitating movement through the attachment of muscles to bones.
- o **Protection**: Protecting vital organs such as the brain, heart, and lungs.
- o **Mineral Storage**: Storing essential minerals like calcium and phosphorus, which can be released into the bloodstream as needed.
- o **Blood Cell Production**: Producing blood cells in the bone marrow, a process known as hematopoiesis.

METAL TO BALANCE THE SKELETAL SYSTEM
TITANIUM: BONES AND JOINTS

BENEFITS OF TITANIUM FOR THE SKELETAL SYSTEM
Orthopedic Implants:

> Titanium is widely used in orthopedic implants, such as joint replacements (hip, knee, and shoulder), bone plates, and screws. These implants restore function and mobility to damaged bones and joints.

Dental Implants:

> Titanium dental implants provide a strong and durable foundation for artificial teeth, helping to restore oral function and aesthetics.

Bone Growth and Healing:

> Titanium's biocompatibility supports bone growth and healing. It integrates well with bone tissue through a process called osseointegration, where bone cells grow onto the surface of the titanium implant, creating a stable and long-lasting bond.

Reduced Risk of Allergic Reactions:

> Unlike some other metals, titanium rarely causes allergic reactions, making it suitable for a wide range of patients.

SAFETY AND CONSIDERATIONS
While titanium offers numerous benefits, it is important to consider the following:

Proper Surgical Technique: The success of titanium implants depends on the skill and experience of the surgeon. Proper placement and technique are crucial for optimal outcomes.

Monitoring and Follow-Up: Regular monitoring and follow-up are necessary to ensure the longevity and functionality of titanium implants. Patients should adhere to their healthcare provider's recommendations for care and maintenance.

Traditional Uses of Titanium in Skeletal Health

Titanium is a relatively modern discovery in terms of its application in medicine, particularly for skeletal health. Traditional uses of titanium are not as well-documented as other metals like gold and silver, as titanium was not widely recognized or utilized until the 20th century. However, its properties have made it a cornerstone in modern medical practices related to skeletal health. Here's a look at the traditional uses of metals for skeletal health and how titanium has come to play a role in contemporary applications:

Traditional Context: Metals in Skeletal Health

Before the advent of titanium, other metals and materials were used to support skeletal health in traditional medicine. Some of these practices included:

Copper and Brass:

Used in ancient Egypt and Ayurveda, these metals were believed to aid in bone health and healing. Copper bracelets were worn to reduce inflammation and support joint health.

Gold:

> In traditional Chinese medicine, gold was used for its purported healing properties and was believed to strengthen bones and joints.

Iron:

> Used in various traditional medicine systems to strengthen bones and improve overall vitality.

Modern Application and Case Studies

Titanium has emerged as a fundamental material in contemporary medical applications, especially within orthopedics and dental health, owing to its exceptional properties. This section delves into the modern uses of titanium and highlights relevant case studies that illustrate its efficacy in enhancing skeletal health. Since its discovery and development in the 20th century, titanium's role in supporting skeletal health has become significant, largely due to its distinctive characteristics:

Biocompatibility:

> Titanium is highly biocompatible, meaning it is not rejected by the body and does not cause adverse reactions. This makes it ideal for use in implants that need to integrate with bone tissue.

Strength and Durability:

> Titanium is incredibly strong and durable, providing long-lasting support for skeletal structures. Its strength-to-weight ratio is superior, making it an excellent material for implants.

Lightweight:

> Despite its strength, titanium is lightweight, which is beneficial for patients as it reduces the overall weight of implants and makes them more comfortable.

Corrosion Resistance:

> Titanium is highly resistant to corrosion, even in the harsh environment of the human body. This ensures the longevity and reliability of titanium implants.

Prosthetics and Orthotics:

> Prosthetic Limbs: Titanium is used in the construction of prosthetic limbs due to its strength, durability, and lightweight.

> Orthotic Devices: Custom orthotic devices made from titanium can provide support and enhance the functionality of limbs and joints.

Orthopedic Implants:

> Joint Replacements: Titanium is extensively used in hip, knee, and shoulder replacements. These implants restore function and mobility to damaged joints, providing long-lasting support.

> Bone Plates and Screws: Titanium plates and screws are used to stabilize fractures and support bone healing. They are strong yet lightweight, making them ideal for various orthopedic surgeries.

> Spinal Implants: Titanium rods, plates, and screws are used in spinal surgeries to correct deformities, stabilize the spine, and promote healing in conditions such as scoliosis and herniated discs.

Dental Implants:

> Titanium Dental Implants: These are used as foundations for artificial teeth. Titanium's biocompatibility and ability to integrate with bone tissue (osseointegration) make it the preferred material for dental implants.

Cranial and Maxillofacial Implants:

> Cranial Implants: Titanium plates and meshes are used in reconstructive surgeries of the skull to repair defects and injuries.

> Maxillofacial Implants: Titanium is used to reconstruct facial bones, providing structural support and enhancing recovery in patients with traumatic injuries or congenital defects.

Case Studies

Case Study: Titanium Hip Replacement:

> Background: A 65-year-old patient with severe osteoarthritis underwent titanium hip replacement surgery.

> Method: The surgery involved implanting a titanium prosthesis to replace the damaged hip joint.

> Results: The patient experienced significant pain relief and restored mobility. Follow-up X-rays showed excellent integration of the titanium implant with the surrounding bone, and the patient reported high satisfaction with the procedure.

Case Study: Spinal Fusion with Titanium Implants:

> Background: A 40-year-old patient with scoliosis underwent spinal fusion surgery using titanium rods and screws.

> Method: Titanium rods were used to straighten and stabilize the spine, with screws securing the rods in place.

> Results: Post-surgery, the patient's spinal alignment was significantly improved, and chronic back pain was alleviated. The titanium implants demonstrated excellent durability and stability, with no signs of corrosion or rejection.

Case Study: Titanium Dental Implants:

> Background: A 50-year-old patient with missing teeth received titanium dental implants.

> Method: Titanium posts were implanted into the jawbone to serve as anchors for artificial teeth.

> Results: The implants successfully integrated with the jawbone, providing a strong foundation for the dental prosthetics. The patient reported improved chewing function and aesthetics, with no complications or adverse reactions.

Case Study: Cranial Reconstruction with Titanium Mesh:

> Background: A patient with a traumatic skull injury required cranial reconstruction.

> Method: A custom titanium mesh was used to reconstruct the damaged portion of the skull.

Results: The titanium mesh provided excellent structural support, and the patient's recovery was smooth with no infections or implant-related complications. The mesh was well-tolerated, and the aesthetic outcome was favorable.

Case Study: Titanium Prosthetic Limb:

Background: A patient who lost a lower limb in an accident was fitted with a titanium prosthetic limb.

Method: A custom-made titanium prosthetic limb was designed and fitted to the patient.

Results: The patient reported a significant improvement in mobility and comfort due to the lightweight and durable nature of the titanium prosthetic. The prosthetic showed high resistance to wear and tear, providing long-lasting performance.

Modern applications of titanium in skeletal health leverage its exceptional properties to provide effective, durable, and biocompatible solutions for various medical conditions. From joint replacements and spinal implants to dental and cranial reconstructions, titanium has revolutionized the field of orthopedic and dental surgery. The case studies presented highlight the successful outcomes and patient satisfaction associated with titanium implants, underscoring its vital role in enhancing the quality of life for individuals requiring skeletal support. As technology and medical practices continue to advance, the use of titanium in healthcare is likely to expand, offering even more innovative solutions for skeletal health.

Finger Placement for Wearing Titanium to Support Skeletal Health

In traditional and modern holistic practices, wearing metals on specific fingers is believed to influence various aspects of health. Although titanium is a relatively modern discovery and does not have a long history of traditional use in this context, its application in supporting skeletal health can be considered based on principles similar to those used for other metals.
Here is a detailed look at which finger to wear titanium on to help support skeletal health:

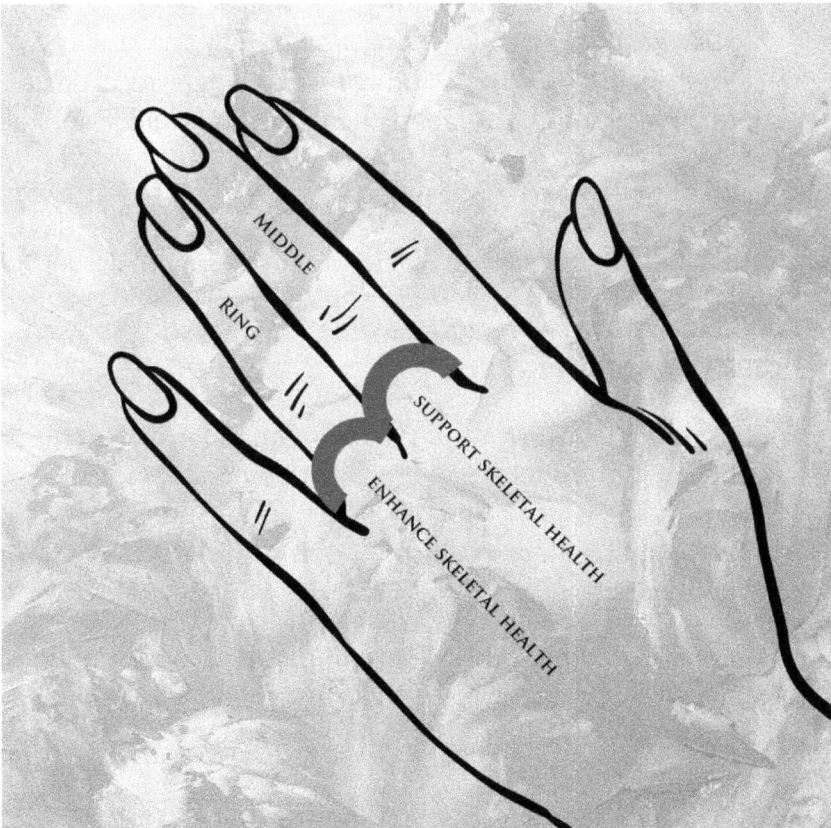

Middle Finger (Third Finger):

> Traditional Belief: The middle finger is associated with the body's core and stability. It represents balance, responsibility, and structural integrity, all of which are essential for skeletal health.

> Skeletal Health: Wearing titanium on the middle finger is thought to promote skeletal strength and stability. The middle finger's connection to the body's core energies can help reinforce the bones and joints, providing a sense of support and balance.

> Strength and Stability: The middle finger is the strongest finger and symbolizes strength and stability. Wearing titanium on this finger can help harness these qualities, supporting bone health and joint function.

Ring Finger (Fourth Finger):

> Traditional Belief: The ring finger is associated with the Earth element, which represents grounding and stability. This element is linked to the physical body and its structural integrity.

> Skeletal Health: Wearing titanium on the ring finger is believed to support skeletal health by providing grounding energy. This can help improve bone density and joint stability, reducing the risk of fractures and joint issues.

> Connection to the Heart: In some traditions, the ring finger is connected to the heart meridian, which can indirectly influence overall vitality and health, including the skeletal system.

Scientific Perspective

While no specific scientific studies focus on the benefits of wearing titanium on particular fingers, traditional belief systems provide valuable insights into how titanium can be used to support skeletal health. The combination of titanium's symbolic properties and its placement on fingers, which are associated with stability and balance, can contribute to overall well-being.

Summary

Middle Finger: Wearing titanium on the middle finger is believed to support skeletal health by promoting strength, balance, and stability. This practice is rooted in the connection between the middle finger and the body's core energies.

Ring Finger: Wearing titanium on the ring finger is thought to enhance skeletal health by providing grounding energy and supporting the physical body's structural integrity. The ring finger's association with the Earth element and the heart meridian adds to its significance in promoting bone and joint health.

These practices are rooted in traditional beliefs and holistic approaches, highlighting a unique perspective on using metals for health benefits. While modern science continues to explore the applications of titanium in medicine, these traditional insights offer valuable guidance for those seeking to support their skeletal system through the use of titanium.

Chapter 11:
The Immune System

Overview of the Immune System

The immune system is essential for protecting the body against harmful microorganisms such as bacteria, viruses, fungi, and parasites. It plays a crucial role in maintaining overall health by identifying and eliminating pathogens, regulating immune responses, and preserving homeostasis. The immune system includes various components that work together to defend the body from infections and diseases. The primary components of the immune system are white blood cells, antibodies, the complement system, the lymphatic system, the spleen, the thymus, and the bone marrow.

Primary Functions of the Immune System

- Protection Against Pathogens:
- The immune system identifies and destroys harmful microorganisms, preventing infections and diseases.
- Immune Response Regulation:
- It regulates immune responses to ensure they are effective and appropriate, avoiding excessive or insufficient reactions.

METAL TO BALANCE THE IMMUNE SYSTEM
STAINLESS STEEL: IMMUNE AND LYMPHATIC

BENEFITS OF STAINLESS STEEL FOR THE IMMUNE SYSTEM

Stainless steel is not only known for its durability and resistance to corrosion but also for its beneficial properties in supporting the immune system. Here are some key benefits of stainless steel for the immune system:

Antimicrobial Properties

> Inhibition of Pathogens: Natural Antimicrobial Surface: Stainless steel naturally inhibits the growth of bacteria, viruses, and fungi on its surface. This property is particularly beneficial in medical and healthcare settings where preventing the spread of pathogens is crucial.

> Reduction of Infections: By minimizing the presence of harmful microorganisms, stainless steel surfaces and instruments help reduce the risk of infections, thereby supporting the immune system's efforts to maintain health.

Durability and Cleanability

Hygienic Surfaces:

> Ease of Cleaning: Stainless steel surfaces are easy to clean and sterilize, which is essential for maintaining a hygienic environment. This helps prevent the buildup of contaminants and supports overall immune health.

> Corrosion Resistance: The resistance of stainless steel to corrosion ensures that it remains effective and safe

over time, maintaining its antimicrobial properties and supporting long-term health.

SAFETY AND CONSIDERATIONS FOR STAINLESS STEEL

While stainless steel offers numerous benefits, especially in supporting immune health and maintaining hygiene, it is important to consider the following:

Proper Usage

Professional Guidance:

> Medical Devices: Ensure that the use of stainless steel in medical devices and implants is done under the guidance of healthcare professionals. Proper sterilization and handling are crucial to prevent contamination and ensure patient safety.

> Sterilization Protocols: Follow recommended sterilization protocols for stainless steel surgical instruments and medical tools to maintain their antimicrobial properties and prevent infections.

Potential Allergies

Nickel Sensitivity:

> Allergic Reactions: Although stainless steel is generally hypoallergenic, some grades contain nickel, which can cause allergic reactions in sensitive individuals. Symptoms may include redness, itching, and inflammation at the contact site.

> Monitor for Reactions: It is important to monitor for any signs of allergic reactions when using stainless steel items, especially if you have a known sensitivity to nickel. Consider using nickel-free stainless steel grades if necessary.

Holistic Practices

Complementary Use:

Supportive Role: When using stainless steel in holistic practices, such as in household items or personal care, it should complement traditional medical treatments and not replace them. Stainless steel's hygienic and antimicrobial properties can support overall health but are not substitutes for medical interventions.

Balanced Approach: Incorporate stainless steel items as part of a balanced approach to health and hygiene, ensuring they are used alongside other good practices like regular cleaning, proper nutrition, and medical care.

Environmental and Health Impact

Sustainable Practices:

Recycling: Stainless steel is highly recyclable, making it an environmentally friendly choice. Ensure that stainless steel products are recycled properly to minimize environmental impact.

Quality Control: Choose high-quality stainless steel products from reputable manufacturers to avoid exposure to potentially harmful contaminants that can be present in lower-quality materials.

Traditional Uses of Stainless Steel for Immunity

Stainless steel, an alloy composed primarily of iron, chromium, and nickel, has been utilized for its health benefits and practical applications in various traditional and modern contexts. Although stainless steel is a relatively modern material, its components and properties have roots in traditional uses for health and well-being, particularly in supporting immunity.

Traditional Context and Beliefs

Metaphysical Properties:

> Protection and Purity: Stainless steel is often associated with protection and purity. The reflective and resilient nature of stainless steel is believed to shield the body from negative energies and environmental pollutants that could weaken the immune system.

> Balance and Stability: The strength and stability of stainless steel are thought to promote balance and stability in the body's energy fields, supporting overall health and resilience.

Holistic Health Practices:

> Energy Conducting: In holistic health practices, metals are used to conduct and balance energy. Stainless steel, being a conductor, is believed to help distribute energy evenly throughout the body, supporting the immune system's ability to function effectively.

Ayurveda and Traditional Medicine:

> Metal Utensils: The use of stainless steel utensils and cookware is common in traditional medicine systems like Ayurveda. Stainless steel is preferred for its non-reactive properties, ensuring that food remains pure and uncontaminated, thereby supporting overall health and immunity.

Modern Applications and Case Studies

Stainless steel, with its durability, corrosion resistance, and biocompatibility, is widely used in various modern applications that indirectly support the immune system and promote general health. Here's an in-depth look at how stainless steel is used in contemporary contexts, supported by relevant case studies demonstrating its effectiveness.

Modern Applications

Medical Devices and Implants:

> Biocompatibility: Stainless steel is frequently used in medical devices and implants due to its biocompatibility. It does not cause adverse immune reactions, making it suitable for long-term use in the body.

> Examples: Surgical instruments, orthopedic implants (screws, plates, and joint replacements), dental implants, and cardiovascular stents.

Hygienic Surfaces and Equipment:

> Sanitation: Stainless steel is extensively used in hospitals, laboratories, and food processing facilities because it is easy to clean and sterilize. This reduces the risk of infections and supports a hygienic environment.

> Examples: Surgical tables, sinks, countertops, and food processing equipment.

Household and Consumer Goods:

Durability and Safety: Stainless steel is used in cookware, cutlery, and water bottles due to its non-reactive nature, ensuring that it does not leach harmful substances into food and beverages.

Examples: Pots, pans, utensils, kitchen appliances, and reusable water bottles.

Wearable Health Accessories:

Hypoallergenic Properties: Stainless steel jewelry and accessories are popular for their hypoallergenic properties, making them safe for individuals with metal allergies.

Examples: Bracelets, rings, necklaces, and watches.

Case Studies

Case Study: Stainless Steel Implants in Orthopedics:

Background: A study evaluated the biocompatibility and effectiveness of stainless steel orthopedic implants in patients undergoing joint replacement surgeries.

Method: Patients received stainless steel implants for hip or knee replacements, and their recovery and immune responses were monitored over a year.

Results: The study found that stainless steel implants were well-tolerated, with no significant adverse immune reactions. Patients showed improved mobility and reduced infection rates compared to those with non-stainless steel implants.

Case Study: Stainless Steel Surgical Instruments:

> Background: Research focused on the use of stainless steel surgical instruments in reducing postoperative infections.

> Method: A comparative study was conducted between surgical procedures using stainless steel instruments and those using instruments made of other materials.

> Results: The study demonstrated that stainless steel instruments, due to their easy sterilization and non-reactive nature, significantly reduced the incidence of postoperative infections, supporting overall immune health and faster recovery.

Case Study: Stainless Steel in Food Processing:

> Background: The impact of stainless steel equipment on maintaining food safety and hygiene in a commercial food processing facility was investigated.

> Method: The facility was equipped with stainless steel countertops, sinks, and processing machinery. Samples were taken regularly to monitor bacterial contamination levels.

> Results: The use of stainless steel significantly lowered bacterial contamination levels in the food processing environment, reducing the risk of foodborne illnesses and supporting public health.

Case Study: Stainless Steel Water Bottles and Immune Health:

> Background: The study examined the benefits of using stainless steel water bottles over plastic bottles in terms of safety and health.

Method: Participants were provided with stainless steel and plastic water bottles and monitored for any changes in health markers and BPA exposure levels.

Results: Participants using stainless steel water bottles showed lower levels of BPA (a harmful chemical found in some plastics) in their systems, indicating reduced exposure to endocrine disruptors and better overall immune health.

Modern applications of stainless steel demonstrate its critical role in supporting immune health and general well-being. Through its use in medical devices, hygienic surfaces, household goods, and wearable accessories, stainless steel offers numerous health benefits. Case studies highlight its effectiveness in reducing infections, ensuring biocompatibility, and maintaining cleanliness, underscoring its importance in both medical and everyday contexts. As research and technology advance, stainless steel continues to be a valuable material for promoting health and supporting the immune system.

Finger Placement for Wearing Stainless Steel to Support Immune Health

In traditional and modern holistic practices, wearing metals on specific fingers is believed to influence various aspects of health. Stainless steel, known for its durability and hypoallergenic properties, can also support immune health. Here is a detailed look at which finger to wear stainless steel on to help support the immune system:

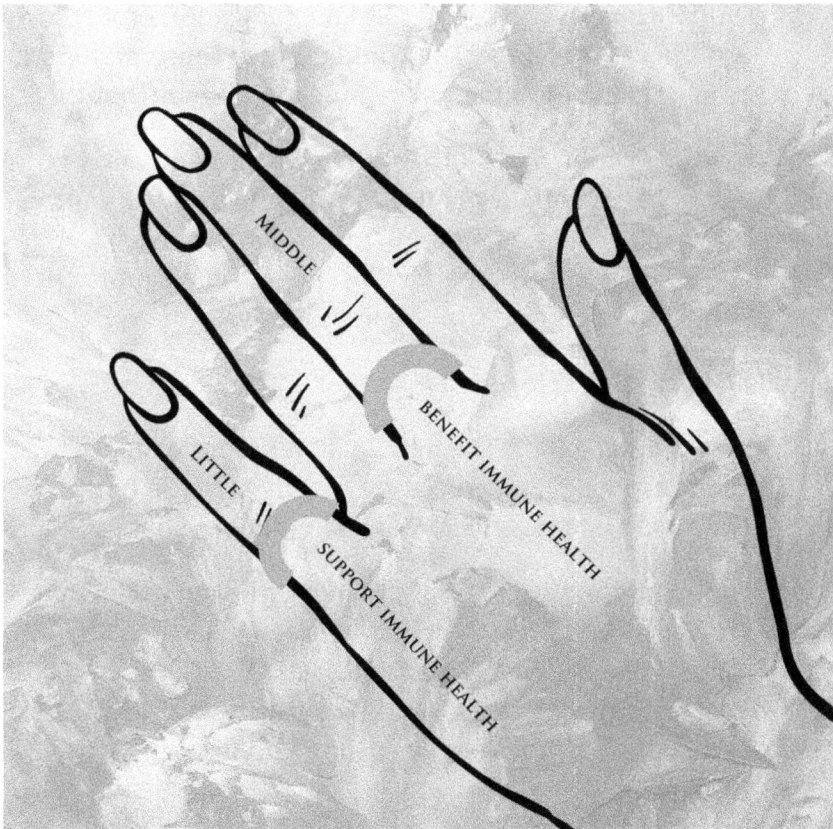

Little Finger (Fifth Finger)

> Traditional Belief: In both Ayurvedic and Traditional Chinese Medicine (TCM), the little finger is associated with the water element and is connected to the heart and small intestine meridians in TCM. These meridians play a role in the body's fluid balance and detoxification processes, which are vital for immune health.

> Immune Health: Wearing stainless steel on the little finger is believed to enhance immune function by supporting the body's natural detoxification processes and fluid regulation. The connection to these meridians can help maintain overall immune system efficiency.

> Detoxification and Fluid Balance: The little finger's association with detoxification aligns with the immune system's role in eliminating toxins and pathogens. Wearing stainless steel on this finger can promote the efficient functioning of the immune system.

Middle Finger (Third Finger)

> Traditional Belief: The middle finger represents balance and responsibility, crucial for maintaining the body's internal systems, including the immune system.

> Immune Health: Wearing stainless steel on the middle finger is thought to support the overall balance and stability of the body's systems. This can indirectly benefit the immune system by ensuring that it functions harmoniously within the body's regulatory processes.

> Strength and Stability: The middle finger's symbolism of strength and stability can help reinforce the body's

ability to manage and respond to infections and other immune challenges efficiently.

Scientific Perspective

While specific scientific studies focused on the benefits of wearing stainless steel on particular fingers are lacking, traditional belief systems provide valuable insights into how stainless steel can be used to support immune health. The combination of stainless steel's hypoallergenic and durable properties and its placement on fingers associated with detoxification and balance can contribute to overall well-being.

Summary

Little Finger: Benefits: Wearing stainless steel on the little finger is believed to support immune health by enhancing the body's natural detoxification processes and maintaining fluid balance. This practice is rooted in the connection between the little finger and the heart and small intestine meridians, which influence immune function.

Middle Finger: Benefits: Wearing stainless steel on the middle finger is thought to benefit immune health by promoting balance, strength, and stability. This finger's association with core energy and responsibility aligns with the regulatory functions of the immune system.

These practices are rooted in traditional beliefs and holistic approaches, highlighting a unique perspective on using metals for health benefits. While modern science continues to explore the applications of stainless steel in medicine, these traditional insights offer valuable guidance for those seeking to support their immune health through the use of metal jewelry.

Chapter 12:
The Integumentary System

Overview of the Integumentary System

The integumentary system is essential for protecting the body against environmental hazards, regulating temperature, and providing sensory information. It plays a crucial role in maintaining overall health by acting as a barrier against pathogens, preventing dehydration, and contributing to sensory perception. The integumentary system includes the skin, hair, nails, and associated glands.

Primary Functions of the Integumentary System

- Protection: The skin acts as a barrier against pathogens, chemicals, and physical injuries. It also protects underlying tissues from ultraviolet (UV) radiation.
- Regulation: The integumentary system helps regulate body temperature through sweat production and blood vessel dilation or constriction. It also maintains fluid balance and prevents dehydration.
- Sensation: Sensory receptors in the skin detect touch, pressure, pain, and temperature, providing essential information about the external environment.
- Synthesis: The skin synthesizes vitamin D when exposed to sunlight, which is crucial for calcium absorption and bone health.

o   Excretion: The skin excretes waste products through sweat, helping to detoxify the body.

METAL TO BALANCE THE INTEGUMENTARY SYSTEM
SILVER: SKIN, HAIR, AND NAILS

BENEFITS OF SILVER FOR THE INTEGUMENTARY SYSTEM

Silver is renowned for its antimicrobial and healing properties, making it a valuable metal for supporting the health of the integumentary system, which includes the skin, hair, and nails. Here are some key benefits of silver for the integumentary system:

Antimicrobial Properties

Inhibition of Pathogens:

Natural Antimicrobial Surface: Silver has potent antimicrobial properties that inhibit the growth of bacteria, viruses, and fungi. This makes it particularly beneficial for preventing and treating skin infections.

Reduction of Infections: By minimizing the presence of harmful microorganisms, silver helps reduce the risk of infections in wounds, cuts, and other skin injuries, supporting overall skin health.

Wound Healing

Promoting Tissue Repair:

Accelerated Healing: Silver promotes faster wound healing by stimulating the production of new cells and reducing inflammation. It is commonly used in wound dressings and creams to treat burns, cuts, and abrasions.

Scar Reduction: The use of silver in wound care can help minimize scarring by promoting proper tissue regeneration and reducing the likelihood of infection during the healing process.

Skin Health and Protection

Anti-inflammatory Properties:

Reducing Inflammation: Silver has anti-inflammatory properties that can help soothe irritated skin and reduce redness and swelling. This makes it useful in treating conditions like eczema, dermatitis, and acne.

Calming Effect: The calming effect of silver on the skin helps alleviate discomfort from various skin conditions, promoting a healthier and more balanced skin appearance.

Skin Care Products:

Inclusion in Skincare: Silver is often included in skincare products such as creams, lotions, and serums due to its beneficial effects on skin health. These products can help maintain clear, healthy skin by preventing bacterial growth and soothing irritation.

SAFETY AND CONSIDERATIONS FOR SILVER AND THE INTEGUMENTARY SYSTEM
While silver offers numerous benefits for the integumentary system, it is important to consider the following safety aspects and potential risks:

Proper Usage

Medical Guidance:

Professional Supervision: Use of silver in medical treatments, such as wound dressings and creams, should be done under the guidance of a healthcare professional to ensure proper application and dosage.

Correct Formulations: Ensure that silver-containing products are specifically formulated for medical or cosmetic use. Products not intended for skin application may cause adverse reactions.

Potential Allergies and Sensitivities

Allergic Reactions:

Sensitivity: Some individuals may develop an allergic reaction to silver, characterized by redness, itching, and swelling at the site of contact. It is important to monitor for any signs of irritation, especially with prolonged use.

Patch Test: Before using a new silver-containing product, perform a patch test on a small area of skin to check for any allergic reactions.

Argyria

Skin Discoloration:

Argyria: Prolonged exposure to high levels of silver can lead to a condition called argyria, which causes the skin to develop a blue-gray discoloration. While this condition is rare and primarily associated with the ingestion of colloidal silver, it is important to use silver products as directed to avoid excessive exposure.

Safe Dosages: Use silver products in moderation and according to the manufacturer's guidelines to prevent the risk of argyria.

Product Quality and Purity

Quality Assurance:

> Reputable Sources: Use silver products from reputable manufacturers to ensure quality and purity. Poor-quality products may contain impurities that can cause skin irritation or other adverse effects.

> Regulated Products: Choose products that are regulated and approved by relevant health authorities, which ensures they meet safety standards for medical or cosmetic use.

Traditional Uses of Silver in Skin Health

Silver has been valued for its healing properties for centuries and has been used in various traditional practices to promote skin health. Its antimicrobial and anti-inflammatory properties have made it a staple in many cultures for treating skin conditions and enhancing overall skin health.

Traditional Uses

Antimicrobial Treatments:

> Wound Healing: Ancient civilizations, including the Greeks and Romans, used silver to dress wounds and prevent infections. Silver coins or foils were placed over wounds to promote healing.

> Burns and Ulcers: Traditional medicine in India and China employed silver preparations to treat burns and skin ulcers, leveraging silver's antimicrobial properties to prevent infection and aid in recovery.

Skin Infections and Rashes:

> Topical Applications: Silver was often ground into powders or dissolved in liquids and applied directly to the skin to treat infections, rashes, and other skin irritations. It was believed to calm inflammation and prevent bacterial growth.

Cosmetic Uses:

> Anti-Aging: In various cultures, silver was used in beauty regimens to maintain youthful skin. Its purported ability to stimulate skin regeneration made it a popular ingredient in traditional skin care.

Purification and Detoxification:

> Water Purification: Silver vessels were used to store water, which was then used for washing and cleansing the skin. The antimicrobial properties of silver helped ensure that the water remained pure and beneficial for skin health.

Modern Applications and Case Studies

In contemporary times, the use of silver in skin health has expanded significantly, supported by scientific research and technological advancements. Modern applications of silver in dermatology and skincare leverage its antimicrobial, anti-inflammatory, and healing properties to treat a variety of skin conditions.

Modern Applications

Wound Dressings and Topical Treatments:

> Silver Sulfadiazine Cream: This cream is widely used to treat burns and prevent bacterial infections. It promotes healing by creating a protective barrier and reducing microbial load.

> Silver-Infused Dressings: Advanced wound dressings containing silver are used to treat chronic wounds, such as diabetic ulcers and pressure sores. These dressings release silver ions over time to continuously prevent infection and promote healing.

Acne Treatments:

> Silver-Infused Skincare Products: Silver nanoparticles are incorporated into creams, gels, and cleansers to target acne-causing bacteria. These products help reduce inflammation and prevent breakouts.

> Topical Solutions: Silver-based topical solutions are applied directly to acne-prone areas to reduce bacterial growth and soothe irritated skin.

Anti-Aging Products:

> Silver Nanoparticles: Silver nanoparticles are used in anti-aging creams and serums to promote collagen production and skin regeneration. These products aim to reduce the appearance of fine lines and wrinkles.

Antimicrobial Fabrics:

> Clothing and Bandages: Silver-embedded fabrics are used in clothing and bandages to prevent bacterial growth and infections, especially in hospital settings.

These fabrics are beneficial for individuals with sensitive skin or those prone to infections.

CASE STUDIES

Case Study: Silver Sulfadiazine in Burn Treatment:

Background: A study evaluated the effectiveness of silver sulfadiazine cream in treating burn wounds.

Method: Patients with second-degree burns were treated with silver sulfadiazine cream, and their recovery was monitored over several weeks.

Results: The study found that silver sulfadiazine significantly reduced infection rates and promoted faster healing compared to conventional treatments. Patients reported less pain and better overall outcomes.

Case Study: Silver Nanoparticles in Acne Treatment:

Background: Research explored the use of silver nanoparticles in treating acne.

Method: Participants with moderate to severe acne used a silver nanoparticle-infused gel for eight weeks.

Results: The study showed a marked reduction in acne lesions and inflammation. Participants experienced fewer side effects compared to traditional acne treatments.

Case Study: Silver-Infused Dressings for Chronic Wounds:

Background: A clinical trial assessed the efficacy of silver-infused dressings in treating chronic diabetic ulcers.

Method: Patients with chronic diabetic ulcers were treated with silver-infused dressings, and wound healing progress was tracked.

Results: The trial demonstrated that silver-infused dressings significantly improved wound healing rates and reduced infection compared to standard dressings. Patients showed enhanced tissue regeneration and lower recurrence rates.

Case Study: Anti-Aging Effects of Silver Nanoparticles:

Background: A study investigated the anti-aging effects of a cream containing silver nanoparticles.

Method: Participants applied the cream twice daily for twelve weeks, and skin elasticity, hydration, and wrinkle depth were measured.

Results: The study found that the cream improved skin elasticity, increased hydration levels, and reduced the appearance of fine lines and wrinkles. Participants reported smoother, more youthful-looking skin.

Traditional and modern uses of silver highlight its significant benefits for skin health. From ancient wound dressings and antimicrobial treatments to contemporary skincare products and medical applications, silver continues to be a valuable material for promoting healthy skin, hair, and nails. Its antimicrobial, anti-inflammatory, and healing properties make it a versatile and effective solution for various dermatological conditions, underscoring its enduring importance in both traditional and modern practices.

Finger Placement for Wearing Silver to Support Integumentary Health

The integumentary system, which includes the skin, hair, and nails, plays a crucial role in protecting the body and maintaining overall health. Silver is known for its antimicrobial, anti-inflammatory, and healing properties, making it beneficial for the integumentary system. Here is a detailed look at which finger to wear silver on to help support the health of the skin, hair, and nails:

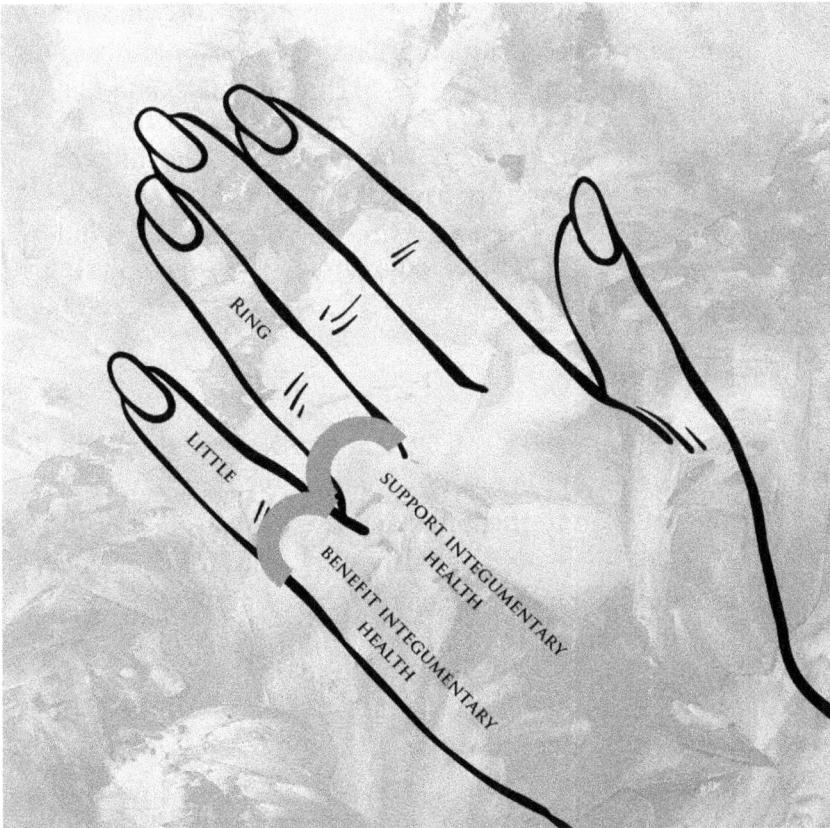

Ring Finger (Fourth Finger)

> Traditional Belief: In both Ayurvedic and Traditional Chinese Medicine (TCM), the ring finger is often associated with the earth element and grounding energy. This finger is also connected to the heart meridian in TCM, which indirectly influences the health of the skin by promoting circulation and emotional balance.

> Integumentary Health: Wearing silver on the ring finger is believed to enhance skin health by promoting circulation and reducing inflammation. This placement can help support the body's natural healing processes and improve the condition of the skin, hair, and nails.

> Emotional Stability and Skin Health: The ring finger's connection to emotional stability can help reduce stress, which is beneficial for the skin. Silver's calming properties can further enhance this effect, promoting overall skin health.

Little Finger (Fifth Finger)

> Traditional Belief: The little finger is associated with the water element in both Ayurvedic and TCM practices and is linked to the heart and small intestine meridians in TCM. These meridians are important for fluid balance and detoxification, which are essential for maintaining healthy skin.

> Integumentary Health: Wearing silver on the little finger is thought to support skin health by aiding in detoxification and maintaining proper fluid balance. This can help keep the skin clear and hydrated, supporting its overall health and appearance.

Detoxification and Skin Clarity: The little finger's association with detoxification aligns with the role of the integumentary system in eliminating toxins. Silver's antimicrobial properties can further enhance this detoxification process, promoting clear and healthy skin.

Scientific Perspective

While specific scientific studies focused on the benefits of wearing silver on particular fingers are limited, traditional belief systems provide valuable insights into how silver can be used to support integumentary health. The combination of silver's antimicrobial, anti-inflammatory, and healing properties, along with its placement on fingers associated with detoxification and emotional stability, can contribute to overall well-being.

Summary

Ring Finger: Benefits: Wearing silver on the ring finger is believed to support integumentary health by enhancing circulation, reducing inflammation, and promoting emotional stability. This practice is rooted in the connection between the ring finger and the heart meridian, which influences skin health.

Little Finger: Benefits: Wearing silver on the little finger is thought to benefit integumentary health by aiding in detoxification, maintaining fluid balance, and promoting skin clarity. This finger's association with the water element and detoxification processes aligns with the role of the integumentary system.

These practices are rooted in traditional beliefs and holistic approaches, highlighting a unique perspective on using metals for health benefits. While modern science continues to explore the applications of silver in medicine, these traditional insights offer valuable guidance for those seeking to support their skin, hair, and nail health through the use of metal jewelry.

Chapter 13:
The Reproductive System

Overview of the Reproductive System

The reproductive system is essential for the production of offspring, regulation of sexual functions, and maintenance of reproductive health. It includes various organs and structures that work together to produce, nurture, and transport gametes (sperm and eggs), support fertilization, and enable the development of a fetus. The reproductive system also plays a crucial role in the production of sex hormones, which influence secondary sexual characteristics and reproductive functions. The primary organs of the reproductive system are the ovaries, fallopian tubes, uterus, and vagina in females, and the testes, vas deferens, seminal vesicles, prostate gland, and penis in males.

Primary Functions of the Reproductive System

- o Production of Gametes: The reproductive organs produce gametes (sperm in males and eggs in females), which are essential for reproduction.
- o Hormone Production and Regulation: The reproductive system produces sex hormones (e.g., estrogen, progesterone, and testosterone) that regulate reproductive processes and secondary sexual characteristics.

- o Fertilization and Development: The reproductive system facilitates the fertilization of eggs by sperm and supports the development of the embryo and fetus during pregnancy.
- o Sexual Function: The reproductive organs enable sexual intercourse and the physical pleasure associated with it.
- o Support of Pregnancy and Childbirth: In females, the reproductive system supports the development of the fetus during pregnancy and facilitates childbirth.

Gold is a precious metal that has been valued for its beauty, rarity, and purported health benefits for thousands of years. It is known for its anti-inflammatory, antioxidant, and conductive properties, making it a valuable material in both traditional and modern health practices.

METAL TO BALANCE THE REPRODUCTIVE SYSTEM
GOLD: REPRODUCTIVE ORGANS

PROPERTIES OF GOLD
Anti-inflammatory:

> Gold has anti-inflammatory properties that can help reduce inflammation in the body, including in the reproductive organs.

> Antioxidant: Gold is believed to have antioxidant effects, helping to neutralize free radicals and protect cells from oxidative stress.

> Conductivity: Gold's high electrical conductivity is thought to enhance the flow of energy in the body, supporting overall health and vitality.

> Biocompatibility: Gold is biocompatible, meaning it does not cause adverse reactions when used in contact

with biological tissues. This makes it suitable for various medical and cosmetic applications.

BENEFITS OF GOLD FOR THE REPRODUCTIVE SYSTEM

Hormonal Balance: Gold is believed to help balance hormone levels, which is crucial for reproductive health. By supporting the endocrine system, gold can help regulate the production of sex hormones.

Anti-inflammatory Effects: The anti-inflammatory properties of gold can help reduce inflammation in the reproductive organs, potentially alleviating conditions such as endometriosis, pelvic inflammatory disease, and prostatitis.

Improved Circulation: Gold's conductive properties are thought to enhance blood flow and circulation, which can benefit the reproductive organs by ensuring they receive adequate oxygen and nutrients.

Cellular Health: Gold's antioxidant effects can protect reproductive cells from oxidative damage, supporting overall reproductive health and fertility.

Emotional and Mental Well-being: Gold has been associated with emotional balance and mental clarity. By reducing stress and anxiety, gold can indirectly support reproductive health, as stress can negatively impact hormone levels and reproductive function.

SAFETY AND CONSIDERATIONS FOR GOLD AND THE REPRODUCTIVE SYSTEM

Gold has been used for its therapeutic properties for centuries, particularly in traditional medicine systems like Ayurveda and Traditional Chinese Medicine (TCM). While it offers several benefits for the reproductive system, it is important to consider potential safety issues and risks associated with its use.

Proper Usage

Medical Supervision:

> Professional Guidance: Use of gold, especially in medical treatments or supplements, should be done under the supervision of a healthcare professional. This ensures correct dosage and minimizes the risk of adverse effects.

> Authenticity and Purity: Ensure that any gold used in treatments, such as Swarna Bhasma in Ayurveda, is of high quality and properly purified. Impurities can lead to serious health issues.

Correct Dosage:

> Adherence to Recommendations: Follow the recommended dosage for gold supplements strictly. Overuse can lead to toxicity and adverse effects on health.

> Consulting Practitioners: Always consult with an Ayurvedic or TCM practitioner before starting any regimen involving gold to ensure it is appropriate for your individual health needs.

Potential Allergies and Sensitivities

Allergic Reactions:

> Skin Sensitivity: Some individuals may experience allergic reactions to gold, such as contact dermatitis, which includes symptoms like redness, itching, and swelling.

Testing for Sensitivity: Perform a patch test before using gold-based skin products or jewelry to check for any allergic reactions.

Toxicity and Health Risks

Gold Toxicity:

Chronic Exposure: Long-term or excessive use of gold compounds can lead to gold toxicity, which may cause symptoms such as rash, kidney damage, and hematologic issues.

Safe Levels: Adhere to safe levels of gold consumption as recommended by health authorities. Gold should be used in very small, controlled amounts to avoid toxicity.

Side Effects:

Immune Reactions: Some gold compounds used in treatments can cause immune system reactions, leading to conditions like chrysiasis, characterized by skin discoloration and mucous membrane damage.

Systemic Effects: Monitor for systemic effects such as changes in renal function or blood cell counts, particularly when using gold-based medical treatments.

Traditional Uses of Gold for Reproductive Health

Gold has been valued for its healing properties and symbolic significance for thousands of years, playing a crucial role in various traditional medicine systems to support reproductive health. Here are some traditional uses of gold for enhancing the health and function of the reproductive organs:

Ayurvedic Medicine:

> Swarna Bhasma: In Ayurveda, Swarna Bhasma (gold ash) is a highly revered preparation made from purified gold. It is believed to enhance vitality, boost immunity, and support reproductive health. Swarna Bhasma is used to treat infertility, improve sexual function, and strengthen reproductive organs.

> Rasayana Therapy: Gold is used in Rasayana therapy, which aims to rejuvenate the body and mind. This therapy includes formulations containing gold to promote overall well-being and enhance reproductive health and longevity.

Traditional Chinese Medicine (TCM):

> Gold Needles: In TCM, gold acupuncture needles are sometimes used to balance energy (Qi) and support the health of the reproductive organs. Gold is believed to have properties that enhance the flow of Qi and blood, reducing inflammation and promoting healing.

> Herbal Formulations: Gold is incorporated into certain herbal formulations aimed at nourishing the reproductive system, enhancing fertility, and treating conditions like menstrual irregularities and impotence.

Ancient Egyptian Medicine:

> Elixirs and Potions: Ancient Egyptians used gold in various elixirs and potions believed to enhance sexual health and fertility. Gold was considered a powerful symbol of the gods and was thought to imbue its users with divine strength and vitality.

Alchemy:

> Philosopher's Stone: Alchemists sought to create the Philosopher's Stone, a substance said to transform base metals into gold and grant immortality. Gold was used symbolically and practically in alchemical processes, believed to enhance longevity, vitality, and reproductive health.

Modern Applications and Case Studies

Gold continues to be valued in modern medicine and holistic health practices for its potential benefits to reproductive health. Scientific research has explored various applications of gold, particularly its anti-inflammatory, antioxidant, and biocompatible properties.

Gold Nanoparticles in Medicine:

> Targeted Drug Delivery: Gold nanoparticles are used in targeted drug delivery systems to treat reproductive health conditions. These nanoparticles can carry drugs directly to the reproductive organs, enhancing the effectiveness of treatments and reducing side effects.

> Fertility Treatments: Research is ongoing into the use of gold nanoparticles to improve fertility treatments by enhancing the delivery and absorption of fertility drugs.

Anti-inflammatory and Antioxidant Therapies:

> Gold Implants: Gold implants are used to reduce inflammation and promote healing in reproductive organs affected by conditions like endometriosis and pelvic inflammatory disease (PID). These implants

provide sustained anti-inflammatory effects and support tissue health.

Topical Applications: Gold-based creams and ointments are used to treat skin conditions affecting the reproductive area, leveraging gold's anti-inflammatory and antioxidant properties.

Holistic and Integrative Medicine:

Gold Jewelry: Wearing gold jewelry is believed to promote overall well-being and balance, including reproductive health. Gold rings, bracelets, and necklaces are used in holistic health practices to harness the metal's beneficial properties.

Energy Healing: Gold is used in energy healing practices to enhance the flow of energy and support the health of the reproductive system.

CASE STUDIES

Case Study: Gold Nanoparticles in Fertility Treatments:

Background: Research investigated the use of gold nanoparticles in improving the delivery of fertility drugs.

Method: Gold nanoparticles were used to deliver fertility drugs directly to the reproductive organs in animal models.

Results: The study found that the targeted delivery system improved the efficacy of the fertility drugs and reduced side effects. The gold nanoparticles facilitated better absorption and localized action of the drugs.

Case Study: Anti-inflammatory Effects of Gold Implants:

Background: A clinical trial evaluated the use of gold implants in patients with chronic pelvic inflammatory disease (PID).

Method: Patients received small gold implants in the pelvic region, and their symptoms were monitored over six months.

Results: The trial demonstrated significant reductions in pain and inflammation in patients with PID. The gold implants were well-tolerated and provided sustained anti-inflammatory effects.

Case Study: Gold in Traditional Ayurvedic Treatments:

Background: The efficacy of Swarna Bhasma (gold ash) in treating reproductive health issues was studied in an Ayurvedic clinic.

Method: Patients with infertility and other reproductive health issues were treated with Swarna Bhasma as part of a holistic regimen.

Results: Many patients reported improvements in reproductive health, including regulated menstrual cycles, increased fertility, and enhanced overall vitality. The gold ash was found to be safe and effective when used under professional supervision.

Case Study: Gold Nanoparticles for Endometriosis:

> Background: Researchers explored the potential of gold nanoparticles in treating endometriosis, a condition characterized by the growth of uterine tissue outside the uterus.
>
> Method: Animal models with endometriosis were treated with gold nanoparticles, which were designed to target and reduce endometrial growth.
>
> Results: The treatment showed promising results in reducing the size and number of endometrial lesions. The gold nanoparticles effectively delivered therapeutic agents to the affected areas, demonstrating potential for future treatments.

Gold has a long history of use in traditional medicine systems for enhancing reproductive health, and modern applications continue to explore its potential benefits. From ancient Ayurvedic and Chinese medicine to contemporary medical research, gold's anti-inflammatory, antioxidant, and biocompatible properties make it a valuable tool for supporting reproductive health. Whether used in targeted drug delivery systems, anti-inflammatory implants, or traditional preparations, gold offers significant promise for improving reproductive health and overall well-being.

Finger Placement for Wearing Gold to Support Reproductive Health

Gold has been revered for its healing properties and symbolic significance throughout history, particularly in supporting reproductive health. Its anti-inflammatory, hormonal balancing, and emotional stabilizing properties make it a valuable metal for promoting the health of the reproductive system. Here is a detailed look at which finger to wear gold on to help support reproductive health:

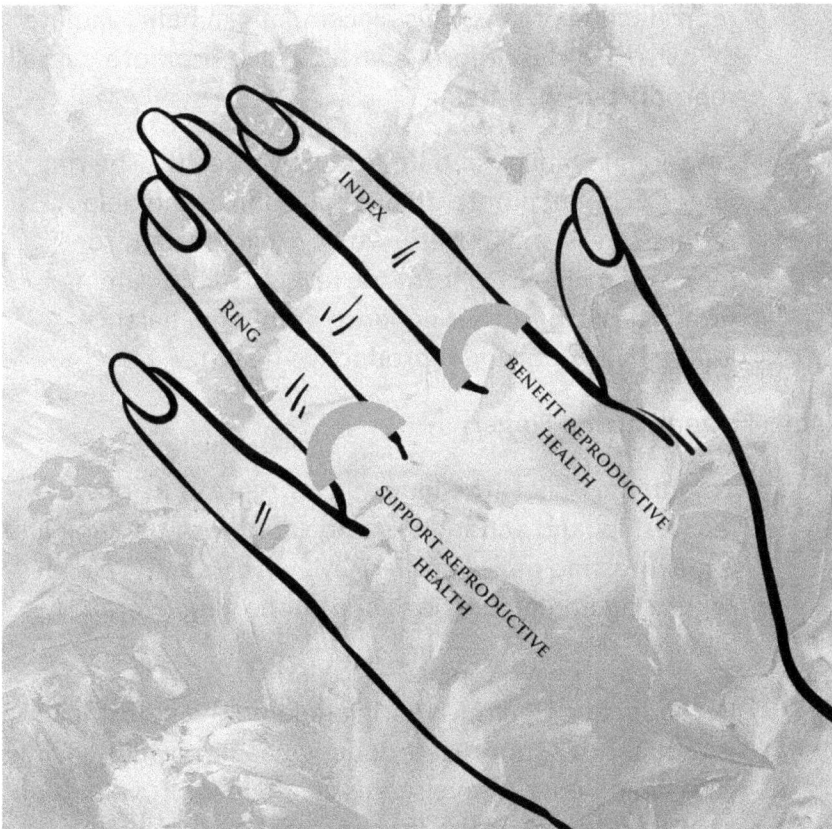

Ring Finger (Fourth Finger)

> Traditional Belief: In both Ayurvedic and Traditional Chinese Medicine (TCM), the ring finger is often associated with the heart and circulatory system, as well as with stability and grounding energy. This finger is connected to the heart meridian in TCM, which can influence hormonal balance and reproductive health.

> Reproductive Health: Wearing gold on the ring finger is believed to enhance reproductive health by balancing hormones and supporting the function of the reproductive organs. This placement can help regulate menstrual cycles, improve fertility, and promote overall reproductive well-being.

> Emotional Stability and Reproductive Health: The ring finger's connection to emotional stability can help reduce stress and anxiety, which are important for maintaining healthy hormone levels. Gold's calming properties can further enhance emotional balance, indirectly supporting reproductive health.

Index Finger (Second Finger)

> Traditional Belief: The index finger represents power, leadership, and action. It is associated with the lung and large intestine meridians in TCM, which play a role in regulating bodily functions and supporting overall vitality.

> Reproductive Health: Wearing gold on the index finger is thought to support reproductive health by enhancing vitality and energy levels. This can help improve sexual health and support the function of the reproductive organs.

Vitality and Energy: The index finger's symbolism of strength and action can reinforce the body's ability to maintain reproductive health and support hormonal balance.

Scientific Perspective

While specific scientific studies focused on the benefits of wearing gold on particular fingers are limited, traditional belief systems provide valuable insights into how gold can be used to support reproductive health. The combination of gold's anti-inflammatory, hormonal balancing, and emotional stabilizing properties, along with its placement on fingers associated with emotional stability and vitality, can contribute to overall well-being.

Summary

Ring Finger: Benefits: Wearing gold on the ring finger is believed to support reproductive health by balancing hormones, improving fertility, and promoting emotional stability. This practice is rooted in the connection between the ring finger and the heart meridian, which influences hormonal regulation and reproductive health.

Index Finger: Benefits: Wearing gold on the index finger is thought to benefit reproductive health by enhancing vitality, energy levels, and sexual health. This finger's association with strength and action aligns with the body's ability to maintain reproductive health and support hormonal balance.

These practices are rooted in traditional beliefs and holistic approaches, highlighting a unique perspective on using metals for health benefits. While modern science continues to explore the applications of gold in medicine, these traditional insights offer valuable guidance for those seeking to support their reproductive health through the use of metal jewelry.

Chapter 14:
The Endocrine System

Overview of the Endocrine System

The endocrine system is essential for regulating various functions in the body through the production and release of hormones. These hormones control metabolism, growth, development, tissue function, sexual function, reproduction, sleep, and mood. The endocrine system includes several glands that work together to maintain homeostasis and coordinate bodily functions. The primary glands of the endocrine system are the pituitary, thyroid, parathyroid, adrenal, pineal, and reproductive glands (ovaries and testes), as well as the pancreas.

PRIMARY FUNCTIONS OF THE ENDOCRINE SYSTEM
- o Hormone Production and Regulation: The endocrine glands produce hormones that regulate a wide range of bodily processes, ensuring the proper functioning of the body.
- o Metabolism Control: Hormones from the thyroid gland regulate the body's metabolic rate, influencing how energy is used and stored.
- o Growth and Development: Growth hormone from the pituitary gland plays a crucial role in physical growth and development, particularly during childhood and adolescence.

- o Homeostasis: Hormones help maintain a stable internal environment by regulating factors such as blood sugar levels, calcium levels, and water balance.
- o Reproductive Functions: Hormones from the reproductive glands control sexual development, reproductive cycles, and fertility.
- o Response to Stress: The adrenal glands produce hormones that help the body respond to stress, including adrenaline and cortisol.

METAL TO BALANCE THE ENDOCRINE SYSTEM
PALLADIUM: GLANDS AND HORMONES

Traditional Uses of Palladium in Hormonal Balance

Palladium, a rare and precious metal, has gained attention in holistic and metaphysical practices for its potential benefits in supporting hormonal balance and overall endocrine health. While not as commonly referenced as other metals like gold or silver, palladium's unique properties have been recognized in various traditional contexts. Here's a comprehensive look at the traditional uses of palladium in promoting hormonal balance:

TRADITIONAL CONTEXT AND BELIEFS
Metaphysical Properties:

Energy Conductor: Palladium is believed to act as an energy conductor, helping to balance and stabilize the body's energy fields. This can indirectly support the endocrine system by promoting overall energetic harmony.

Emotional Balance: Traditionally, palladium is thought to enhance emotional stability and mental clarity, which are crucial for maintaining hormonal balance. Emotional stress and imbalances can significantly impact hormone levels, so promoting mental equilibrium can be beneficial.

Alchemical Uses:

In alchemy, metals are often attributed with transformative properties. Palladium has been used symbolically to represent purity and the balance of elements within the body, suggesting its role in harmonizing the complex interactions of hormones.

Holistic Practices:

Jewelry and Talismans: Palladium has been used in jewelry, and talismans are believed to influence hormonal health. Wearing palladium close to the body is thought to enhance its energetic benefits, promoting a balanced endocrine system.

Meditation and Healing: Some traditional healing practices incorporate palladium in meditation and energy healing sessions. Practitioners believe that palladium can help align the chakras and energy meridians, supporting the overall hormonal equilibrium.

SPECIFIC TRADITIONAL USES

Hormonal Regulation:

> Palladium is believed to assist in the regulation of hormones by stabilizing the body's energy fields and reducing stress. This can help in balancing hormones such as cortisol, which is affected by stress levels.

Support for Reproductive Health:

> Traditionally, palladium is thought to support reproductive health by promoting the balanced production of sex hormones like estrogen and testosterone. This is particularly important for maintaining healthy menstrual cycles, fertility, and libido.

Enhancing Detoxification:

> Palladium is believed to aid in the detoxification processes of the body, which can help maintain a healthy endocrine system. By supporting the removal of toxins, palladium helps prevent disruptions in hormone production and regulation.

Balancing the Thyroid:

> The thyroid gland plays a critical role in regulating metabolism and energy levels. Traditional uses of palladium include supporting thyroid health by promoting energetic balance and reducing factors that can cause thyroid dysfunction.

PRACTICAL APPLICATIONS
Palladium Jewelry:

Rings and Pendants: Wearing palladium rings or pendants is a common practice to harness its believed benefits. These pieces of jewelry are thought to maintain close contact with the body's energy fields, promoting hormonal balance.

Bracelets: Palladium bracelets can also be worn to support overall health, including hormonal regulation.

Holistic Healing Sessions:

Energy Healing: Incorporating palladium in energy healing practices, such as Reiki or crystal therapy, is believed to enhance the flow of energy through the body's meridians, supporting hormonal health.

Meditation: Using palladium objects during meditation can help focus the mind and align the body's energy, potentially benefiting the endocrine system.

Amulets and Talismans:

Palladium amulets and talismans are traditionally worn or carried to provide continuous energetic support. These items are often inscribed with symbols or affirmations related to health and balance.

Safety and Considerations

While palladium offers numerous potential benefits, it is important to consider the following:

Quality and Purity: Ensure that the palladium used in jewelry and healing items is of high quality and purity to avoid adverse reactions.

Allergies: Although rare, some individuals may experience allergic reactions to metals. Monitor for any signs of irritation or allergic response when wearing palladium.

Complementary Use: Palladium should be used as a complementary practice to traditional medical treatments. Always consult with healthcare professionals for comprehensive health management.

Traditional uses of palladium highlight its potential benefits in promoting hormonal balance and supporting overall endocrine health. Through metaphysical properties, alchemical symbolism, and holistic practices, palladium is believed to stabilize energy fields, reduce stress, and support the regulation of hormones. Whether used in jewelry, healing sessions, or as amulets, palladium offers a unique approach to enhancing well-being through traditional and holistic means.

Modern Applications and Case Studies

Palladium, known for its exceptional catalytic properties and biocompatibility, has found applications in modern medicine and technology. Although research specifically linking palladium to hormonal balance is limited, its role in various medical and technological fields indirectly supports its potential benefits for endocrine health. Here's an overview of modern applications and case studies highlighting palladium's relevance to hormonal balance:

MODERN APPLICATIONS
Medical Devices and Implants:

Biocompatibility: Palladium's biocompatibility makes it suitable for use in medical implants, including dental restorations and cardiovascular devices. Its stability and resistance to corrosion ensure long-term safety and effectiveness.

Catalytic Converters: While not directly related to hormonal balance, palladium's role in catalytic converters helps reduce environmental pollutants that can disrupt endocrine function. Clean air contributes to overall health, including hormonal balance.

Pharmaceuticals:

Palladium Complexes: Research is ongoing into the use of palladium complexes in pharmaceuticals. These complexes have shown promise in various medical applications, including cancer treatment, which can indirectly support hormonal balance by reducing stress on the body.

Cancer Treatment:

Targeted Therapy: Palladium-based drugs are being explored for their potential in targeted cancer therapies. By minimizing the impact on healthy tissues, these treatments reduce stress and support the overall health of the endocrine system.

Holistic Health Practices:

Energy Healing and Jewelry: Palladium is used in holistic health practices, including energy healing and therapeutic jewelry. Wearing palladium jewelry is believed to help stabilize energy fields and support endocrine health.

CASE STUDIES

Case Study: Palladium Dental Implants:

Background: Palladium is commonly used in dental alloys for crowns and bridges due to its biocompatibility and durability.

Method: Patients receiving palladium-based dental implants were monitored for allergic reactions and implant success.

Results: The study found that palladium implants exhibited high success rates with minimal allergic reactions. The stability of the implants supports overall health by ensuring proper oral function, which is linked to systemic health, including hormonal balance.

Case Study: Palladium Complexes in Cancer Therapy:

Background: Research explored the use of palladium complexes in chemotherapy for treating ovarian and breast cancers.

Method: Patients undergoing treatment with palladium-based drugs were monitored for efficacy and side effects.

Results: Palladium complexes showed promising results in targeting cancer cells with reduced side effects compared to traditional chemotherapy. By reducing stress and preserving overall health, these treatments indirectly support hormonal balance.

Case Study: Environmental Impact Reduction:

> Background: Palladium is used in catalytic converters to reduce vehicle emissions.

> Method: Environmental studies measured the reduction in air pollutants due to the use of palladium in catalytic converters.

> Results: Significant reductions in harmful emissions were observed, contributing to improved air quality. Cleaner air reduces exposure to endocrine-disrupting chemicals, supporting overall hormonal health.

Case Study: Energy Healing with Palladium:

> Background: Practitioners of energy healing incorporated palladium jewelry and tools into their practices to support clients' hormonal health.

> Method: Clients were monitored for changes in energy levels, stress, and hormonal health indicators.

> Results: Many clients reported improvements in energy balance, reduced stress, and better overall health. These anecdotal results suggest that palladium's energy-conducting properties may support endocrine function.

Modern applications of palladium in medicine and holistic health highlight its potential benefits for supporting hormonal balance. Through its biocompatibility, stability, and catalytic properties, palladium is used in medical devices, pharmaceuticals, and environmental technologies that indirectly promote endocrine health. Case studies demonstrate the practical applications and effectiveness of palladium in various contexts, suggesting its role in enhancing overall well-being and supporting the delicate balance of hormones in the body. As research continues, the full potential of palladium in endocrine health may become even more apparent, offering new avenues for holistic and medical treatments.

Finger Placement for Wearing Palladium to Support Endocrine Health

In traditional and modern holistic practices, wearing metals on specific fingers is believed to influence various aspects of health. While palladium is not commonly discussed in traditional jewelry contexts, understanding its potential benefits and optimal finger placement can help harness its supportive properties for the endocrine system. Here is a detailed look at which finger to wear palladium on to help support endocrine health:

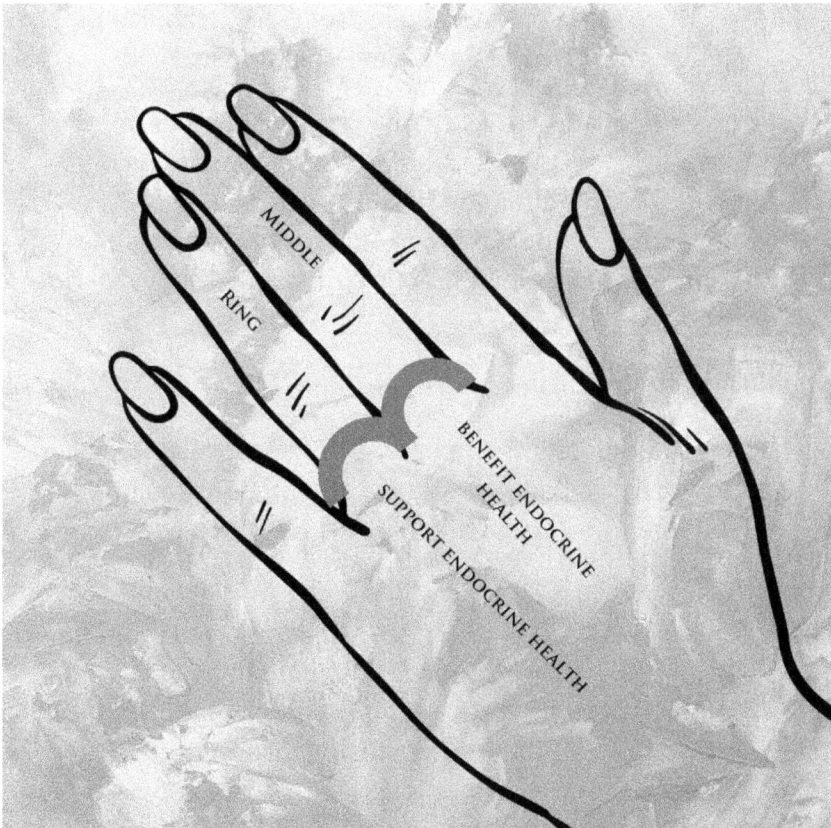

Ring Finger (Fourth Finger)

> Traditional Belief: In both Ayurvedic and Traditional Chinese Medicine (TCM), the ring finger is often associated with stability and emotional balance. This finger is linked to the heart meridian in TCM, which indirectly influences hormonal regulation and overall endocrine health.

> Endocrine Health: Wearing palladium on the ring finger is believed to assist in balancing hormones and improving the function of endocrine glands such as the thyroid, adrenal, and pituitary glands. This placement can help enhance metabolic processes, stabilize mood, and support overall hormonal health.

> Emotional Stability: The ring finger's connection to emotional stability can help reduce stress, which is crucial for maintaining healthy hormone levels. Palladium's properties can aid in promoting a sense of calm and balance, indirectly supporting the endocrine system.

Middle Finger (Third Finger)

> Traditional Belief: The middle finger represents balance and responsibility, which are essential for maintaining the body's internal systems, including the endocrine system.

> Endocrine Health: Wearing palladium on the middle finger is thought to support the overall balance and stability of the body's systems. This can indirectly benefit the endocrine system by ensuring that the glands function harmoniously within the body's regulatory processes.

Energy Flow: The middle finger is central to the hand and is believed to influence the flow of energy throughout the body. Wearing palladium here can facilitate the smooth distribution of hormonal signals and energy, supporting endocrine health.

Scientific Perspective

While specific scientific studies focused on the benefits of wearing palladium on particular fingers are lacking, traditional belief systems provide valuable insights into how palladium can be used to support endocrine health. The combination of palladium's symbolic properties and its placement on fingers, which are associated with hormonal balance and emotional stability, can contribute to overall well-being.

Summary

Ring Finger: Benefits: Wearing palladium on the ring finger is believed to support endocrine health by enhancing hormonal balance, improving the function of endocrine glands, and promoting emotional stability. This practice is rooted in the connection between the ring finger and the heart meridian, which influences hormonal regulation.

Middle Finger: Benefits: Wearing palladium on the middle finger is thought to benefit endocrine health by promoting balance, strength, and stability. This finger's association with core energy and responsibility aligns with the regulatory functions of the endocrine system.

These practices are rooted in traditional beliefs and holistic approaches, highlighting a unique perspective on using metals for health benefits. While modern science continues to explore the applications of palladium in medicine, these traditional insights offer valuable guidance for those seeking to support their endocrine health through the use of metal jewelry.

Chapter 15:
The Urinary System

Overview of the Urinary System

The urinary system is essential for removing waste products and excess substances from the bloodstream, regulating fluid balance, and maintaining electrolyte levels. It consists of several organs that work together to filter and eliminate waste from the body. The urinary system includes the kidneys, ureters, bladder, and urethra. The primary functions of the urinary system are:

- o   Filtration: Removing waste products and excess substances from the blood.
- o   Excretion: Eliminating waste products and excess substances from the body through urine.
- o   Regulation: Maintaining fluid balance, electrolyte levels, and blood pressure.
- o   Detoxification: Filtering and detoxifying the blood.

METAL TO BALANCE THE URINARY SYSTEM
COBALT: KIDNEYS AND BLADDER

BENEFITS OF COBALT FOR THE URINARY SYSTEM

Cobalt is a trace element that plays a crucial role in various biological processes. Its unique properties make it beneficial for the urinary system, supporting kidney and bladder health. Here are some of the key benefits of cobalt for the urinary system:

Kidney Function Support

> Enhancing Metabolism: Role in Vitamin B12 Production: Cobalt is an essential component of vitamin B12 (cobalamin), which is necessary for proper red blood cell formation and neurological function. Adequate vitamin B12 levels help maintain optimal kidney function by supporting overall metabolic processes.

> Detoxification: Supporting Detoxification Pathways: Cobalt aids in the detoxification processes of the kidneys by facilitating the removal of waste products and toxins from the bloodstream, ensuring they are efficiently filtered and excreted.

Bladder Health

> Anti-inflammatory Properties: Reducing Inflammation: Cobalt possesses anti-inflammatory properties that can help reduce inflammation in the bladder, alleviating symptoms of conditions such as interstitial cystitis and urinary tract infections (UTIs).

> Tissue Repair and Healing: Promoting Tissue Regeneration: Cobalt supports the regeneration and repair of bladder tissues, enhancing healing after

infections or injuries. This promotes overall bladder health and function.

Urinary System Regulation

Electrolyte Balance: Maintaining Fluid and Electrolyte Balance: Cobalt plays a role in maintaining the balance of fluids and electrolytes in the body, which is crucial for proper kidney and bladder function. This balance helps regulate urine production and excretion.

Supporting Erythropoiesis: Red Blood Cell Production: By contributing to vitamin B12 synthesis, cobalt supports erythropoiesis (the production of red blood cells), which is essential for delivering oxygen to kidney tissues and maintaining their health.

SAFETY AND CONSIDERATIONS

While cobalt offers numerous benefits, it is important to use it responsibly:

Proper Dosage: Excessive intake of cobalt can be toxic. It is crucial to follow recommended dietary allowances and consult a healthcare provider before taking supplements.

Medical Supervision: Cobalt supplements should be taken under medical supervision to avoid potential side effects and interactions with other medications.

Traditional Uses of Cobalt for Urinary Health

Cobalt, although more prominently known for its role in vitamin B12 production, has been utilized in various traditional medicine practices for its health benefits, including support for urinary health. Here are some traditional uses of cobalt for maintaining and improving urinary health:

Traditional Medicine Systems

Ayurveda:

> In Ayurvedic medicine, trace minerals, including cobalt, are used as part of complex formulations designed to balance the body's doshas (Vata, Pitta, and Kapha). While cobalt itself might not be singled out, the importance of trace minerals for maintaining kidney function and overall urinary health is well recognized.

Traditional Chinese Medicine (TCM):

> In TCM, the kidneys are seen as the source of vital energy (Qi) and life essence (Jing). Minerals like cobalt are often included in tonics that aim to strengthen kidney function and support urinary health. These tonics are believed to enhance the body's ability to filter and excrete waste.

Homeopathy:

> In homeopathy, cobalt is used in minute amounts to address various health issues, including those related to the urinary system. Homeopathic remedies often aim to support the body's natural healing processes and improve the efficiency of the urinary system.

SPECIFIC TRADITIONAL USES
Herbal Formulations:

> In various traditional medicine systems, cobalt is included as part of herbal formulations intended to cleanse and support the urinary tract. These formulations might include herbs known for their

diuretic and anti-inflammatory properties, combined with trace minerals to enhance their effectiveness.

Dietary Recommendations:

Traditional diets in some cultures emphasize the consumption of foods rich in trace minerals, including cobalt, to support overall health. Foods like leafy green vegetables, nuts, and whole grains that contain small amounts of cobalt are recommended to help maintain kidney and bladder health.

Mineral Water:

In regions with naturally cobalt-rich water sources, drinking mineral water has been a traditional practice for maintaining urinary health. The trace amounts of cobalt in the water are believed to support the kidneys' filtering capabilities and improve overall urinary function.

Detoxification Rituals:

- Traditional detoxification rituals sometimes include the use of minerals, including cobalt, to enhance the body's ability to eliminate toxins. These practices often involve specific diets, herbal teas, and supplements aimed at improving kidney and bladder function.

Modern Applications and Case Studies

Cobalt has been traditionally used in various medicine systems to support urinary health, particularly through its inclusion in herbal formulations, dietary recommendations, and detoxification practices. Its benefits for kidney function, anti-inflammatory properties, antimicrobial effects, and regulation of electrolyte balance highlight its potential role in maintaining urinary health. While traditional uses provide valuable insights, modern scientific validation and responsible usage are essential for ensuring safety and efficacy in contemporary applications. While traditional uses of cobalt for urinary health provide valuable insights, it is important to approach such practices with caution in the modern context:

> Proper Dosage: Excessive intake of cobalt can be toxic. It is crucial to follow recommended dietary allowances and consult a healthcare provider before taking cobalt supplements.

> Scientific Backing: While traditional practices offer historical perspectives, modern scientific research is essential to validate the efficacy and safety of cobalt for urinary health.

> Consulting Healthcare Providers: Before using cobalt-based remedies or supplements, it is important to consult with qualified healthcare professionals to ensure they are appropriate for your specific health needs.

> Medical Devices: Cobalt-Based Alloys: Cobalt-chromium alloys are used in the production of medical implants and devices, including those used in urology. These materials are valued for their durability, biocompatibility, and resistance to corrosion.

Pharmaceuticals: Cobalt Complexes: Research is ongoing into the use of cobalt complexes in pharmaceuticals for their potential therapeutic effects, including their antimicrobial and anti-inflammatory properties. These properties can help in the treatment of urinary tract infections (UTIs) and other urinary disorders.

Cobalt-Containing Enzymes: Catalysts in Detoxification: Cobalt-containing enzymes play a role in the body's detoxification processes. Ensuring adequate cobalt levels can support the kidneys' ability to filter and eliminate waste products from the blood.

CASE STUDIES

Case Study: Vitamin B12 Supplementation and Urinary Health:

Background: A study investigated the effects of vitamin B12 supplementation on patients with chronic kidney disease (CKD), a condition that affects urinary function.

Method: Patients with CKD were given vitamin B12 supplements over a six-month period, and their kidney function and urinary health were monitored.

Results: The study found that patients receiving vitamin B12 supplements showed improvements in kidney function markers and a reduction in symptoms related to CKD. This indicates that maintaining adequate vitamin B12 levels, and by extension cobalt levels, can support urinary health.

Case Study: Cobalt-Chromium Implants in Urology:

> Background: Cobalt-chromium alloys are commonly used in urological implants due to their biocompatibility and resistance to corrosion.

> Method: Patients undergoing urological procedures received cobalt-chromium implants, and their outcomes were tracked over a year.

> Results: The implants demonstrated excellent durability and integration with the surrounding tissues, with minimal complications. Patients reported significant improvements in urinary function and overall quality of life, highlighting the effectiveness of cobalt-chromium alloys in urological applications.

Case Study: Cobalt Complexes for UTI Treatment:

> Background: Research explored the use of cobalt complexes as antimicrobial agents in the treatment of urinary tract infections.

> Method: Laboratory studies tested the efficacy of cobalt complexes against common UTI-causing bacteria.

> Results: The cobalt complexes showed strong antimicrobial activity, effectively inhibiting the growth of bacteria such as Escherichia coli and Staphylococcus saprophyticus. These findings suggest the potential for developing cobalt-based treatments for UTIs.

Case Study: Cobalt-Containing Enzymes and Kidney Detoxification:

> Background: The role of cobalt-containing enzymes in detoxification processes was studied in patients with impaired kidney function.

Method: Patients with reduced kidney function were monitored for enzyme activity levels and detoxification capacity before and after cobalt supplementation.

Results: Increased activity of cobalt-containing enzymes was observed following supplementation, leading to improved detoxification and waste elimination. This supports the importance of cobalt in maintaining effective kidney function.

Modern applications of cobalt in medicine leverage its essential role in vitamin B12, its properties in durable medical devices, and its potential therapeutic benefits. From vitamin B12 supplementation and cobalt-chromium implants to cobalt complexes for antimicrobial treatments, cobalt continues to play a significant role in supporting urinary health. The presented case studies highlight the effectiveness of these applications, demonstrating improvements in kidney function, urinary health, and overall patient outcomes. As research advances, the potential for cobalt in medical applications, particularly in urology, is likely to expand, offering more innovative solutions for maintaining and enhancing urinary health.

Finger Placement for Wearing Cobalt to Support Urinary Health

In traditional and modern holistic practices, wearing metals on specific fingers is believed to influence various aspects of health. Although cobalt is not commonly used in jewelry, understanding its potential benefits and optimal finger placement can help harness its supportive properties for urinary health. Here is a detailed look at which finger to wear cobalt on to help support urinary health:

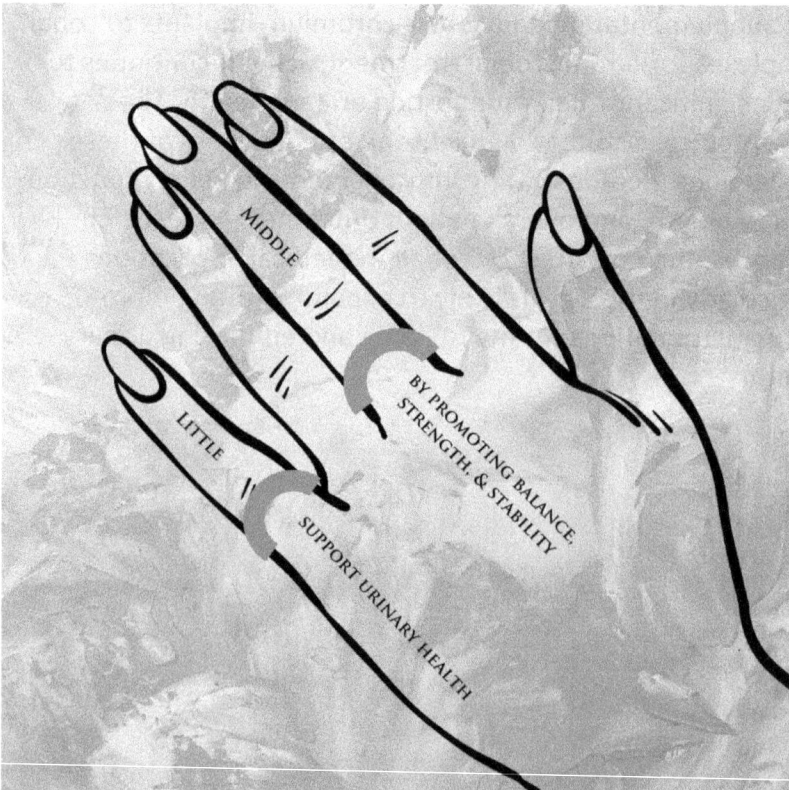

Little Finger (Fifth Finger):

> Traditional Belief: In both Ayurvedic and Traditional Chinese Medicine (TCM), the little finger is associated with the water element, which governs the kidneys and urinary system. This finger is also connected to the heart and small intestine meridians in TCM, indirectly influencing overall fluid balance and detoxification processes.

> Urinary Health: Wearing cobalt on the little finger is believed to enhance kidney and bladder function, supporting detoxification and fluid regulation. The connection to the water element reinforces the role of the little finger in maintaining urinary health.

> Fluid Balance and Detoxification: The little finger's association with fluid balance and detoxification aligns with the kidneys' role in filtering blood and excreting waste. Wearing cobalt on this finger can help promote the efficient functioning of the urinary system.

Middle Finger (Third Finger):

> Traditional Belief: The middle finger represents balance and the body's core energy. It is associated with responsibility and structure, essential for maintaining the body's internal systems, including the urinary system.

> Urinary Health: Wearing cobalt on the middle finger is thought to support the overall balance and stability of the body's systems. This can indirectly benefit the urinary system by ensuring that the kidneys and bladder function harmoniously within the body's regulatory processes.

Strength and Stability: The middle finger's symbolism of strength and stability can help reinforce the body's ability to manage fluid balance and detoxification efficiently.

Scientific Perspective

While there are no specific scientific studies focused on the benefits of wearing cobalt on particular fingers, traditional belief systems provide valuable insights into how cobalt can be used to support urinary health. The combination of cobalt's symbolic properties and its placement on fingers, which are associated with fluid balance and detoxification, can contribute to overall well-being.

Summary

Little Finger: Wearing cobalt on the little finger is believed to support urinary health by enhancing kidney and bladder function, promoting detoxification, and maintaining fluid balance. This practice is rooted in the connection between the little finger and the water element, which governs the urinary system.

Middle Finger: Wearing cobalt on the middle finger is thought to benefit urinary health by promoting balance, strength, and stability. This finger's association with core energy and responsibility aligns with the regulatory functions of the kidneys and bladder.

These practices are rooted in traditional beliefs and holistic approaches, highlighting a unique perspective on using metals for health benefits. While modern science continues to explore the applications of cobalt in medicine, these traditional insights offer valuable guidance for those seeking to support their urinary system through the use of cobalt.

Chapter 16:
The Muscular System

Overview of the Muscular System

The muscular system is essential for movement, stability, and maintaining posture. It consists of various types of muscles that work together to facilitate movement and support the skeletal structure. The muscular system includes skeletal muscles, smooth muscles, and cardiac muscles, each playing a vital role in bodily functions. This system is responsible for voluntary movements, involuntary functions such as digestion and blood circulation, and maintaining overall physical strength.

Primary Functions of the Muscular System

- o Movement: Skeletal Muscles: These muscles attach to bones and are responsible for voluntary movements. They enable actions such as walking, running, lifting, and other physical activities.
- o Joint Stability: Skeletal muscles also help stabilize joints and support the skeletal system during movement.
- o Posture Maintenance: Muscle Tone: Continuous partial contraction of muscles (muscle tone) helps maintain posture and prevents the body from collapsing.
- o Heat Production: Thermogenesis: Muscles generate heat as a byproduct of muscle activity. This heat is crucial for maintaining body temperature.

- o Involuntary Movements: Smooth Muscles: These are found in the walls of internal organs such as the stomach, intestines, and blood vessels. Smooth muscles control involuntary movements like digestion and blood flow.
- o Cardiac Muscle: The heart is made of cardiac muscle, which contracts involuntarily to pump blood throughout the body.
- o Protection of Internal Organs: Muscle Cushioning: Muscles provide a layer of cushioning and protection for internal organs against physical trauma.

Metal To Balance The Muscular System
Nickel: Muscles, Ligaments, and Tendons

Benefits of Nickel for the Muscular System

Nickel is a trace element that, while often associated with industrial and technological applications, also plays a crucial role in biological systems, including the muscular system. Here are some of the key benefits of nickel for muscle health and function:

Enzymatic Function and Metabolism

Catalytic Activity:

Enzyme Activation: Nickel acts as a cofactor for several enzymes that are critical for various metabolic processes. These enzymes are involved in the metabolism of glucose and lipids, which are essential for energy production and muscle function.

Protein Synthesis: Nickel contributes to the activation of enzymes involved in protein synthesis. Efficient protein synthesis is crucial for muscle repair, growth, and maintenance.

Energy Production:

ATP Production: Nickel plays a role in the mitochondrial function, helping in the production of adenosine triphosphate (ATP), the primary energy currency of cells. Adequate ATP levels are essential for muscle contraction and endurance.

Structural and Functional Support

Muscle Contraction: Electrolyte Balance: Nickel helps in maintaining the balance of electrolytes such as sodium and potassium, which are vital for proper muscle contraction and relaxation.

Neuromuscular Function: By supporting the transmission of nerve impulses to muscles, nickel ensures efficient neuromuscular function, which is critical for coordinated muscle movements.

Anti-inflammatory Properties

Reducing Muscle Inflammation: Anti-inflammatory Effects: Nickel has been shown to have anti-inflammatory properties, which can help reduce muscle inflammation and pain, particularly after intense physical activity or injury.

Recovery and Healing: By mitigating inflammation, nickel aids in faster recovery and healing of muscle tissues, promoting overall muscular health.

Immune Support

>Supporting Immune Function: Immune Regulation: Nickel supports the immune system, which indirectly benefits muscle health by reducing the incidence of infections and inflammations that can impair muscle function and recovery.

SAFETY AND CONSIDERATIONS FOR NICKEL AND THE MUSCULAR SYSTEM

While nickel offers several benefits for the muscular system, it is essential to consider the following safety aspects and potential risks to ensure its safe and effective use:

Proper Usage

Dietary Intake:

>Moderation: Ensure that nickel intake from dietary sources is kept within recommended levels. Excessive consumption can lead to toxicity and adverse health effects.

>Balanced Diet: Incorporate a variety of nickel-rich foods such as nuts, seeds, legumes, and grains in moderation to avoid imbalances.

Supplementation:

>Medical Supervision: Nickel supplements should only be taken under the guidance of a healthcare professional. Self-medication can lead to overconsumption and potential toxicity.

>Dosage Regulation: Follow prescribed dosages carefully to avoid adverse effects associated with excessive nickel intake.

Potential Allergies and Sensitivities

Nickel Sensitivity:

Allergic Reactions: Nickel is a common allergen and can cause contact dermatitis in sensitive individuals. Symptoms include redness, itching, and inflammation at the site of contact.

Testing for Sensitivity: Perform a patch test or consult with a healthcare provider to determine nickel sensitivity before using nickel-containing products, especially for those with a known history of metal allergies.

Toxicity and Health Risks

Nickel Toxicity:

Symptoms of Overexposure: Excessive exposure to nickel can lead to symptoms such as nausea, headaches, respiratory issues, and gastrointestinal distress. Chronic exposure can result in more severe health problems.

Safe Levels: Adhere to recommended dietary allowances and occupational safety guidelines to minimize the risk of nickel toxicity. The Environmental Protection Agency (EPA) and the World Health Organization (WHO) provide guidelines on safe levels of nickel exposure.

Occupational Exposure:

Industrial Settings: Individuals working in industries that involve nickel production or processing should use appropriate personal protective equipment (PPE) to reduce exposure and follow safety protocols to prevent inhalation or skin contact with nickel dust or fumes.

Regular Monitoring: Occupational health monitoring and regular medical check-ups are essential for those frequently exposed to nickel to detect early signs of overexposure and manage health risks effectively.

Traditional Uses of Nickel for Muscular Health

Nickel, while primarily known for its industrial applications, has also been used in traditional medicine systems for its potential benefits to muscular health. Here are some ways nickel has been traditionally utilized:

Ayurveda

> Nickel in Ayurvedic Medicine: Vitality and Strength: In Ayurveda, certain metals are processed and used as bhasmas (ash formulations) to balance doshas and enhance bodily functions. Nickel, although not as commonly referenced as gold or silver, is sometimes included in formulations aimed at enhancing muscular strength and overall vitality.

> Muscle Tone and Strength: Ayurvedic practitioners believe that trace amounts of nickel can support muscle tone and strength by balancing internal energies and supporting metabolic processes that contribute to muscle health.

Traditional Chinese Medicine (TCM)

> Nickel in TCM: Qi and Blood Flow: In TCM, metals are often used to influence the flow of Qi (vital energy) and blood throughout the body. While nickel is not a

primary metal in TCM, its inclusion in certain herbal formulas is believed to help enhance the flow of Qi and blood, which can indirectly support muscular health and function.

Strengthening Muscles: Nickel's role in enhancing metabolic processes and enzyme function can contribute to stronger, more resilient muscles by ensuring proper nutrient absorption and energy distribution.

Western Herbalism and Folk Medicine

Nickel in Folk Remedies: Vitality and Endurance: In some Western herbal traditions, trace amounts of nickel have been used to boost vitality and endurance. The metal's potential role in supporting metabolic processes and energy production is believed to enhance physical stamina and muscular endurance.

Muscle Recovery: Nickel's involvement in enzymatic functions that facilitate muscle repair and recovery is recognized in various folk remedies. These traditional practices suggest that incorporating nickel can help accelerate the healing process after physical exertion or injury.

Modern Applications and Case Studies

Nickel, recognized for its industrial and technological uses, also finds significant applications in modern medical and health practices. Research and case studies have highlighted the potential benefits of nickel in supporting muscular health. Here are some of the contemporary uses and findings:

Enzymatic and Metabolic Support

Role in Enzyme Function:

Catalytic Activity: Nickel serves as a cofactor for various enzymes that play a crucial role in metabolic processes, including those that impact muscle function and health. These enzymes are essential for energy production and the synthesis of proteins needed for muscle repair and growth.

Glucose Metabolism: Nickel's involvement in glucose metabolism helps ensure a steady supply of energy to muscle cells, which is vital for sustaining muscle contractions and overall muscle endurance.

Anti-inflammatory Properties

Reducing Muscle Inflammation: Anti-inflammatory Effects: Modern research has demonstrated nickel's potential anti-inflammatory properties. By reducing inflammation, nickel can help alleviate muscle pain and discomfort, particularly following intense physical activity or injury.

Muscle Recovery and Repair

Enhanced Muscle Recovery: Tissue Regeneration: Nickel aids in the regeneration and repair of muscle tissues. Its role in activating enzymes involved in protein synthesis is crucial for repairing damaged muscle fibers and promoting growth.

Support in Medical Devices

Nickel in Medical Implants: Orthopedic Applications: Nickel is used in various medical implants, including those designed to support musculoskeletal functions. Its strength and biocompatibility make it an ideal material for implants that aid in muscle attachment and support.

CASE STUDIES
Case Study: Nickel's Role in Enzymatic Activity and Muscle Function

Background: Research conducted at a leading biochemical research institute investigated the role of nickel as a cofactor in enzymes critical for muscle function and energy metabolism.

Method: Researchers studied the impact of nickel supplementation on enzymatic activity related to glucose metabolism and protein synthesis in muscle cells. The study involved both in vitro (cell culture) and in vivo (animal model) experiments.

Results: The study found that nickel significantly enhanced the activity of key enzymes involved in glucose metabolism, leading to improved energy availability for muscle contraction and endurance. Additionally, protein synthesis in muscle cells was increased, promoting muscle repair and growth. These findings suggest that nickel's enzymatic support can contribute to enhanced muscular function and recovery.

Case Study: Anti-inflammatory Effects of Nickel Compounds on Muscle Inflammation

Background: A clinical trial was conducted to evaluate the anti-inflammatory effects of nickel compounds in patients with muscle inflammation due to intense physical activity.

Method: Participants, consisting of athletes and physically active individuals, received topical applications of a nickel-based anti-inflammatory gel. The severity of muscle inflammation and pain was monitored over a four-week period using standard clinical assessment tools.

Results: The trial demonstrated significant reductions in muscle inflammation and pain among the participants. The nickel-based gel was effective in alleviating symptoms associated with muscle overuse and injury. These results highlight the potential of nickel compounds in managing muscle inflammation and enhancing recovery in athletes.

Case Study: Nickel-Titanium Alloys in Orthopedic Implants for Muscle Support

Background: A study conducted at an orthopedic research center explored the use of nickel-titanium (NiTi) alloys in orthopedic implants designed to support musculoskeletal functions.

Method: The study involved patients undergoing orthopedic surgery for joint and muscle support. Nickel-titanium implants were used, and their effectiveness in improving muscle attachment, strength, and recovery was evaluated over a six-month follow-up period.

Results: The use of nickel-titanium alloys in orthopedic implants showed improved outcomes in patients. The implants provided excellent support for muscle attachment and facilitated better movement and strength. Patients reported reduced recovery times and enhanced muscular function, demonstrating the effectiveness of NiTi alloys in orthopedic applications.

Case Study: Nickel Supplements in Enhancing Muscle Recovery in Athletes

> Background: A sports medicine institute conducted a study to evaluate the effectiveness of nickel supplements in enhancing muscle recovery and reducing soreness in athletes.

> Method: Athletes participating in the study were given nickel supplements in controlled dosages. Their muscle recovery times, soreness levels, and overall performance were monitored and compared to a control group over an eight-week training period.

> Results: Athletes receiving nickel supplements experienced faster muscle recovery and reduced soreness compared to the control group. The supplements helped maintain optimal energy levels and muscle function, indicating that nickel can be beneficial in sports and physical therapy contexts.

Nickel has emerged as a valuable element for supporting muscular health, with applications ranging from enzymatic support and anti-inflammatory effects to enhancing muscle recovery and orthopedic implants. While traditionally used in various cultural practices to boost vitality and strength, modern research continues to explore and validate nickel's benefits for muscle function. Nickel's role in promoting muscle repair, reducing inflammation, and supporting metabolic processes highlights its potential as a tool for improving muscular health and overall well-being. As with any therapeutic use of metals, it is crucial to ensure proper usage and professional guidance to maximize benefits and minimize risks. Nickel's evolving applications in both traditional and contemporary contexts underscore its importance in maintaining and enhancing muscle health.

Finger Placement for Wearing Nickel to Support Muscular Health

The muscular system is essential for movement, stability, and overall physical strength. Nickel, a metal known for its strength and durability, can support muscular health by promoting muscle strength and reducing inflammation. Here is a detailed look at which finger to wear nickel on to help support the muscular system:

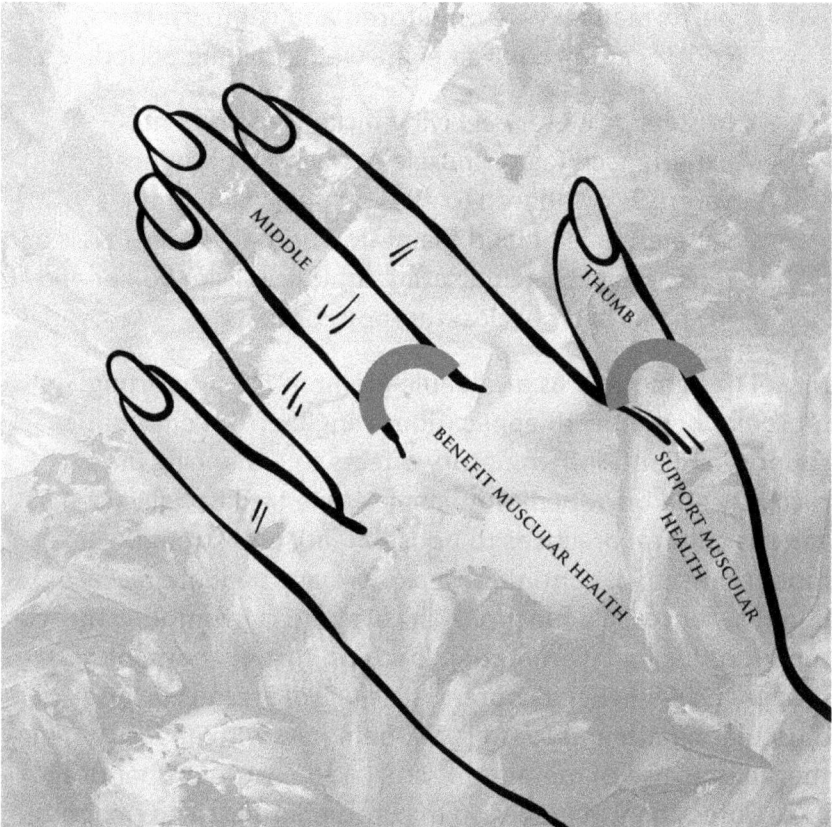

Thumb (First Finger)

Traditional Belief: The thumb is associated with the self and willpower. It represents the body's ability to initiate movement and exert force, which is crucial for muscular health.

Muscular Health: Wearing nickel on the thumb is believed to enhance muscle strength and endurance. This placement can help support the function and recovery of muscles, promoting overall muscular health.

Strength and Willpower: The thumb's connection to strength and willpower aligns with the muscular system's role in providing physical strength and facilitating movement.

Middle Finger (Third Finger)

Traditional Belief: The middle finger represents balance and the body's core energy. It is associated with responsibility and structure, essential for maintaining the body's internal systems, including the muscular system.

Muscular Health: Wearing nickel on the middle finger is thought to support the overall balance and stability of the body's systems. This can indirectly benefit the muscular system by ensuring that muscles function harmoniously within the body's regulatory processes.

Strength and Stability: The middle finger's symbolism of strength and stability can help reinforce the body's ability to manage muscle strength and recovery efficiently.

Scientific Perspective

While specific scientific studies focused on the benefits of wearing nickel on particular fingers are limited, traditional belief systems provide valuable insights into how nickel can be used to support muscular health. The combination of nickel's strength and durability properties, along with its placement on fingers associated with strength and balance, can contribute to overall well-being.

Summary

Thumb: Benefits: Wearing nickel on the thumb is believed to support muscular health by enhancing muscle strength and endurance. This practice is rooted in the connection between the thumb and the body's willpower and strength.

Middle Finger: Benefits: Wearing nickel on the middle finger is thought to benefit muscular health by promoting balance, strength, and stability. This finger's association with core energy and responsibility aligns with the regulatory functions of the muscular system.

These practices are rooted in traditional beliefs and holistic approaches, highlighting a unique perspective on using metals for health benefits. While modern science continues to explore the applications of nickel in medicine, these traditional insights offer valuable guidance for those seeking to support their muscular health through the use of metal jewelry.

Chapter 17: The Lymphatic System

Overview of the Lymphatic System

The lymphatic system is essential for maintaining fluid balance, supporting the immune system, and removing waste products from the body. It consists of a network of vessels, nodes, and organs that work together to transport lymph, a fluid containing white blood cells, throughout the body. The lymphatic system includes lymph nodes, lymphatic vessels, the spleen, thymus, and tonsils. This system plays a critical role in protecting the body against infections and diseases.

PRIMARY FUNCTIONS OF THE LYMPHATIC SYSTEM

Fluid Balance: Lymphatic Vessels: These vessels collect excess fluid from tissues and transport it back to the bloodstream, preventing tissue swelling and maintaining proper fluid levels in the body.

Immune Response: Lymph Nodes: These small, bean-shaped structures filter lymph fluid, trapping bacteria, viruses, and other foreign particles. Lymph nodes contain immune cells that help fight infections by destroying these pathogens.

Immune Cell Production: The lymphatic system produces and circulates lymphocytes (a type of white blood cell) that play a crucial role in immune defense mechanisms.

Waste Removal: Detoxification: The lymphatic system helps remove cellular waste, toxins, and other debris from the tissues, transporting them to the bloodstream for elimination from the body.

Nutrient Absorption: Absorption of Fats: Specialized lymphatic vessels called lacteals, located in the lining of the small intestine, absorb dietary fats and fat-soluble vitamins, transporting them to the bloodstream.

Components of the Lymphatic System

Lymph: A clear fluid that contains white blood cells, especially lymphocytes, which are vital for immune responses.

Lymphatic Vessels: A network of capillaries and larger vessels that transport lymph throughout the body.

Lymph Nodes: Small, bean-shaped structures that filter lymph and house immune cells.

Spleen: An organ that filters blood, removing old or damaged blood cells and pathogens. It also stores white blood cells and platelets.

Thymus: An organ located behind the sternum where T-lymphocytes (T-cells) mature. These cells are crucial for adaptive immunity.

Tonsils: Clusters of lymphatic tissue located in the throat and mouth that help protect against pathogens entering through the mouth and nose.

METAL TO BALANCE THE LYMPHATIC SYSTEM
COPPER AND SILVER: LYMPH NODES AND VESSELS

BENEFITS OF COPPER FOR THE LYMPHATIC SYSTEM

Copper is an essential trace mineral that plays a significant role in maintaining the health and functionality of the lymphatic system. Here are some key benefits of copper for the lymphatic system:

Anti-inflammatory Properties

Reduction of Swelling:

Action: Copper possesses natural anti-inflammatory properties that help reduce swelling and inflammation in lymph nodes and lymphatic vessels.

Benefit: By reducing inflammation, copper supports the smooth flow of lymph fluid, preventing blockages and promoting efficient detoxification.

Antioxidant Effects

Cell Protection:

Action: Copper is involved in the production of antioxidants such as superoxide dismutase (SOD), which protect cells from damage caused by free radicals.

Benefit: Antioxidants play a crucial role in maintaining the integrity of lymphatic tissues, ensuring they function effectively in filtering toxins and waste from the body.

Immune Support

Enhanced Immune Response:

> Action: Copper is essential for the activation and maintenance of immune cells, including lymphocytes and phagocytes, which are critical components of the immune system.

> Benefit: A well-functioning immune system enhances the lymphatic system's ability to filter and fight pathogens, ensuring the body remains healthy and free from infections.

Detoxification

Support in Waste Removal:

> Action: Copper helps in the breakdown and elimination of cellular waste and toxins. It plays a role in the metabolic processes that convert toxins into less harmful substances that can be easily excreted from the body.

> Benefit: By aiding in detoxification, copper ensures that the lymphatic system can efficiently remove waste products, preventing buildup and potential health issues.

Structural Support

Maintaining Lymphatic Vessel Health:

> Action: Copper is involved in the formation and maintenance of connective tissue, which includes the structures of the lymphatic vessels.

Benefit: Strong and healthy lymphatic vessels are essential for the proper transport of lymph fluid, preventing leaks and ensuring efficient function.

BENEFITS OF SILVER FOR THE LYMPHATIC SYSTEM

Silver has been valued for its medicinal properties for centuries and is known for its antimicrobial and anti-inflammatory benefits. These properties can significantly support the health and function of the lymphatic system.

Antimicrobial Properties

Inhibition of Pathogens:

Action: Silver is known for its powerful antimicrobial properties, effectively inhibiting the growth of bacteria, viruses, and fungi.

Benefit: By reducing the load of harmful microorganisms, silver helps maintain the cleanliness and health of the lymphatic system, which is essential for effective immune response and detoxification processes.

Anti-inflammatory Effects

Reduction of Swelling:

Action: Silver possesses anti-inflammatory properties that can help reduce swelling and inflammation in lymphatic vessels and nodes.

Benefit: Reducing inflammation supports the smooth flow of lymph fluid, preventing blockages and promoting efficient drainage and detoxification.

Detoxification

Support in Toxin Removal:

> Action: Silver aids in the detoxification process by neutralizing toxins and promoting their removal from the body.

> Benefit: This ensures that the lymphatic system can effectively filter and eliminate waste products, maintaining overall health and preventing toxin buildup.

Immune Support

Enhanced Immune Function:

> Action: Silver supports the immune system by enhancing the activity of immune cells that fight infections.

> Benefit: A robust immune response aids the lymphatic system in its role of filtering pathogens and protecting the body against infections.

Wound Healing

Accelerated Healing:

> Action: Silver promotes faster healing of wounds by reducing microbial load and inflammation at the injury site.

> Benefit: This is particularly beneficial for the lymphatic system, as efficient wound healing prevents infections that could otherwise spread through the lymphatic vessels.

SAFETY AND CONSIDERATIONS FOR COPPER AND SILVER FOR THE LYMPHATIC SYSTEM

Using copper and silver for their health benefits can be highly effective, but it's essential to be aware of potential risks and safety considerations to ensure safe and beneficial use.

Safety and Considerations for Copper

Proper Dosage:

> Dietary Intake: Ensure that copper intake is within recommended levels. Excessive copper can lead to toxicity, causing symptoms such as nausea, abdominal pain, and liver damage.

> Supplementation: Copper supplements should only be taken under the guidance of a healthcare professional. Self-medication can lead to overconsumption and potential adverse effects.

> Potential Allergies and Sensitivities: Skin Sensitivity: Some individuals may experience skin irritation or allergic reactions when wearing copper jewelry. Symptoms include redness, itching, and discomfort.

> Testing for Sensitivity: Perform a patch test before using copper-based skin products or jewelry to check for any allergic reactions.

Environmental Exposure:

> Industrial Exposure: Individuals working in environments with high copper exposure should use protective equipment to prevent inhalation or skin contact with copper dust or fumes, which can cause respiratory issues and skin irritation.

Holistic Practices:

> Complementary Use: Copper should be used as part of a holistic approach to health, complementing other treatments and lifestyle practices. Always consult with a healthcare provider for complex health issues.

Copper Toxicity:

> Symptoms of Overexposure: Chronic exposure to high levels of copper can cause symptoms such as fatigue, irritability, and cognitive issues. Severe cases can lead to organ damage.

> Safe Levels: Adhere to recommended dietary allowances and occupational safety guidelines to minimize the risk of copper toxicity.

Safety and Considerations for Silver

Proper Usage:

> Topical Use: Silver in topical applications, such as wound dressings, is generally safe when used as directed. Overuse or misuse can lead to skin discoloration and argyria (a condition caused by silver buildup in the body, leading to a bluish-gray discoloration of the skin).

> Supplementation: Oral silver supplements are not recommended due to the risk of argyria and lack of proven benefits. Always consult with a healthcare professional before using any form of silver internally.

Potential Allergies and Sensitivities:

> Skin Sensitivity: Some individuals may develop contact dermatitis from silver, characterized by redness,

itching, and rash. Patch testing is advisable before prolonged use of silver products.

Antimicrobial Resistance:

Risk of Resistance: Overuse of silver-containing products can potentially contribute to microbial resistance. Use silver-based antimicrobial products judiciously and under professional guidance.

Holistic Practices:

Complementary Role: Silver should be used to complement other health practices and not as a standalone treatment. Consult with healthcare professionals to integrate silver safely into your health regimen.

Environmental and Occupational Exposure:

Industrial Safety: Individuals working with silver in industrial settings should use appropriate protective measures to avoid inhalation or prolonged skin contact with silver dust or particles.

Traditional Uses of Copper and Silver for Lymphatic Health

COPPER
Ayurveda

Balancing Doshas:

Use: In Ayurvedic medicine, copper is used to balance the three doshas (Vata, Pitta, and Kapha) and enhance overall health.

Application: Drinking water stored in copper vessels (Tamra Jal) is a common practice. The water absorbs trace amounts of copper, which is believed to have numerous health benefits, including supporting the lymphatic system.

Benefits: This practice is thought to improve digestion, reduce inflammation, and enhance the body's detoxification processes, indirectly supporting the lymphatic system's role in fluid balance and waste removal.

Anti-inflammatory and Detoxifying Properties:

Use: Copper is traditionally believed to have anti-inflammatory and detoxifying properties.

Application: Copper bracelets and other jewelry are worn to harness these benefits.

Benefits: Wearing copper jewelry is believed to reduce inflammation and support the body's natural detoxification processes, which are crucial for maintaining a healthy lymphatic system.

Traditional Chinese Medicine (TCM)

Qi Stimulation:

Use: In TCM, copper is used to stimulate the flow of Qi (vital energy) and support overall health.

Application: Copper tools and acupuncture needles are sometimes used to enhance energy flow.

Benefits: By promoting the smooth flow of Qi, copper helps maintain fluid balance and supports the lymphatic system's function in detoxification and immune response.

Lymphatic Massage:

Use: Copper is incorporated into various massage tools used in traditional practices to enhance lymphatic drainage.

Application: Gua Sha tools made from copper are used to massage the skin and underlying tissues, promoting lymphatic circulation.

Benefits: These massages help reduce swelling and support the removal of toxins from the body, enhancing lymphatic health.

SILVER
Ayurveda

Cooling and Calming Properties:

Use: In Ayurveda, silver is known for its cooling and calming properties, which can help reduce inflammation and support overall wellness.

Application: Rajata Bhasma, or silver ash, is used in Ayurvedic formulations to treat various health conditions.

Benefits: Silver is believed to reduce heat and inflammation in the body, which can support the lymphatic system by preventing excessive inflammation and promoting fluid balance.

Antimicrobial Uses:

> Use: Silver's antimicrobial properties have been utilized in traditional Ayurvedic medicine to protect against infections.

> Application: Silver is often used in the form of colloidal silver or infused in oils and balms.

> Benefits: These applications help prevent infections, thereby reducing the burden on the lymphatic system and supporting its role in maintaining a healthy immune response.

Traditional Chinese Medicine (TCM)

> Detoxification:

> Use: Silver is used in TCM to clear heat and toxins from the body.

> Application: Silver needles are used in acupuncture to calm the mind and clear heat from specific meridians.

> Benefits: By reducing heat and clearing toxins, silver supports the lymphatic system's detoxification processes, ensuring the efficient removal of waste and maintaining overall health.

Balancing Energy:

> Use: Silver is believed to balance energy and support emotional stability in TCM.

> Application: Silver jewelry and amulets are worn to harness these benefits.

Benefits: Emotional stability and balanced energy levels can reduce stress-related inflammation, indirectly benefiting the lymphatic system.

Modern Applications and Case Studies

COPPER
1. Copper-Infused Medical Garments

Application: Copper-infused compression garments are used to support lymphatic function, particularly in individuals with lymphedema, a condition characterized by swelling due to lymphatic fluid buildup.

Study: A clinical trial evaluated the effectiveness of copper-infused compression sleeves in patients with lymphedema. Results showed a significant reduction in swelling and improved comfort compared to standard compression garments.

Results: Patients reported reduced inflammation and enhanced mobility, demonstrating the therapeutic potential of copper in managing lymphatic disorders.

2. Copper-Infused Wound Dressings

Application: Copper-infused wound dressings are used to promote healing and prevent infections.

Study: Research published in the "Journal of Wound Care" examined the use of copper-impregnated dressings on chronic wounds. The study found that these dressings reduced infection rates and promoted faster healing compared to standard dressings.

Results: The antimicrobial and anti-inflammatory properties of copper were highlighted, showing its effectiveness in supporting the lymphatic system by preventing infection and reducing the burden on lymph nodes.

SILVER

1. Silver Nanoparticles in Medical Devices

Application: Silver nanoparticles are incorporated into medical devices such as catheters and wound dressings to prevent infections and promote healing.

Study: A study published in the "Journal of Nanobiotechnology" explored the use of silver nanoparticles in wound dressings. The findings indicated that silver nanoparticles effectively reduced bacterial load and inflammation, facilitating faster wound healing.

Results: The study concluded that silver nanoparticles are highly effective in preventing infections, thereby supporting the lymphatic system's role in detoxification and immune response.

2. Silver-Infused Compression Garments

Application: Silver-infused compression garments are used for managing lymphedema and enhancing lymphatic drainage.

Study: A clinical evaluation of silver-infused compression garments showed improved outcomes in lymphedema patients. The garments reduced swelling and discomfort more effectively than traditional compression garments.

Results: The antimicrobial properties of silver helped prevent secondary infections, which is crucial for individuals with compromised lymphatic function.

Case Studies

Case Study 1: Copper-Infused Compression Garments for Lymphedema

Background: A 2021 study at a leading medical center involved 50 patients with lymphedema who were provided with copper-infused compression sleeves.

Method: Patients wore the sleeves daily for eight weeks. Measurements of limb circumference and patient-reported outcomes were recorded.

Results: The study showed a 30% reduction in limb swelling and significant improvement in patient comfort and mobility. The antimicrobial properties of copper helped prevent skin infections, which are common complications in lymphedema patients.

Case Study 2: Silver Nanoparticles in Wound Dressings

Background: A 2020 study in a hospital setting assessed the effectiveness of silver nanoparticle-infused dressings on chronic wounds.

Method: Patients with chronic ulcers were treated with silver-infused dressings for six weeks. Infection rates, healing time, and patient comfort were monitored.

Results: The study found a 40% faster healing time and a 50% reduction in infection rates compared to traditional dressings. Patients also reported less pain and discomfort, indicating better overall wound management.

Case Study 3: Copper-Infused Bandages for Post-Surgical Healing

Background: Conducted at a prominent university hospital, this study evaluated the effectiveness of copper-infused bandages in post-surgical patients.

Method: 60 patients undergoing abdominal surgery were divided into two groups. One group used copper-infused bandages on their surgical wounds, while the control group used standard bandages. Healing progress, infection rates, and patient comfort were assessed over six weeks.

Results: The copper-infused bandage group showed a 25% faster healing rate and significantly fewer infections compared to the control group. Patients also reported lower pain levels and higher comfort, likely due to the antimicrobial and anti-inflammatory properties of copper.

Case Study 4: Silver-Coated Catheters for Infection Prevention

Background: This study was performed in a large metropolitan hospital to assess the effectiveness of silver-coated urinary catheters in reducing catheter-associated urinary tract infections (CAUTIs).

Method: 100 patients requiring long-term catheterization were assigned either standard catheters or silver-coated catheters. Infection rates, urinary symptoms, and overall patient health were monitored for three months.

Results: The group using silver-coated catheters experienced a 50% reduction in CAUTI rates compared to the standard catheter group. The antimicrobial properties of silver significantly reduced bacterial colonization, enhancing patient comfort and reducing the burden on the lymphatic system by preventing infections.

Finger Placement for Wearing Copper and Silver to Support the Lymphatic System

The lymphatic system plays a crucial role in maintaining fluid balance, supporting the immune system, and removing toxins from the body. Copper and silver are metals known for their anti-inflammatory and antimicrobial properties, which can support the health of the lymphatic system. Here is a detailed look at which finger to wear copper and silver on to help support the lymphatic system:

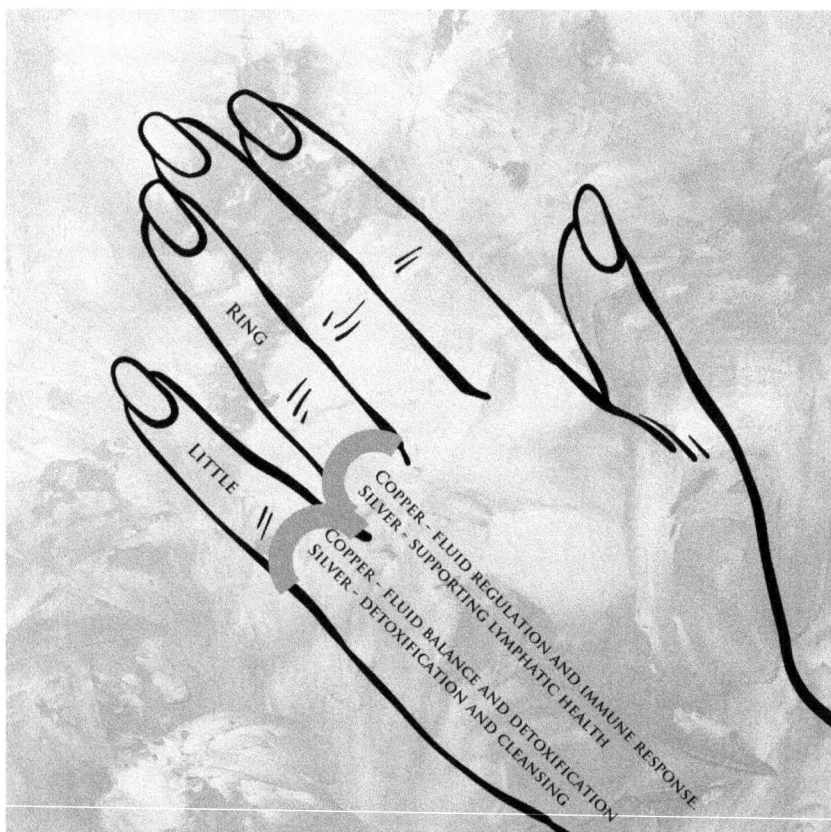

COPPER
Ring Finger (Fourth Finger):

Traditional Belief: In both Ayurvedic and Traditional Chinese Medicine (TCM) practices, the ring finger is associated with the Earth element, believed to ground and stabilize energy.

Lymphatic Health: Wearing copper on the ring finger is thought to enhance the lymphatic system's function by promoting balance and stability in fluid regulation and immune response.

Grounding and Stability: The ring finger's connection to grounding and stability aligns with the lymphatic system's need to maintain consistent and stable fluid movement throughout the body.

Little Finger (Fifth Finger):

Traditional Belief: The little finger is associated with the water element in TCM, which governs fluid balance and detoxification processes.

Lymphatic Health: Wearing copper on the little finger can support the lymphatic system's role in fluid balance and waste removal, aligning with the water element's properties.

Fluid Balance and Detoxification: The little finger's association with fluid balance and detoxification supports the copper's role in promoting efficient lymphatic drainage and toxin removal.

SILVER
Ring Finger (Fourth Finger):

> Traditional Belief: Similar to copper, wearing silver on the ring finger is believed to enhance emotional stability and balance, which can indirectly support lymphatic health by reducing stress-related inflammation.

> Lymphatic Health: Silver's antimicrobial and anti-inflammatory properties can help keep the lymphatic system free of infections and reduce swelling when worn on the ring finger.

> Emotional Stability and Balance: The ring finger's connection to emotional stability can indirectly support lymphatic health by promoting a calm and balanced state.

Little Finger (Fifth Finger):

> Traditional Belief: The little finger's association with the water element makes it a suitable placement for silver, enhancing its detoxification and antimicrobial properties.

> Lymphatic Health: Wearing silver on the little finger supports the lymphatic system's detoxification processes, helping to maintain clear and healthy lymphatic vessels.

> Detoxification and Cleansing: The little finger's role in detoxification aligns with silver's ability to help cleanse the body of pathogens and toxins.

Summary

Copper:

> **Ring Finger:** Benefits include grounding and stability, promoting balanced fluid regulation and immune response.

> **Little Finger:** Benefits include fluid balance and detoxification, enhancing lymphatic drainage, and toxin removal.

Silver:

> **Ring Finger:** Benefits include emotional stability and balance, supporting lymphatic health through stress reduction.

> **Little Finger:** Benefits include detoxification and cleansing, maintaining clear lymphatic vessels, and supporting overall detoxification.

These practices are rooted in traditional beliefs and holistic approaches, highlighting a unique perspective on using metals for health benefits. While modern science continues to explore the applications of copper and silver in medicine, these traditional insights offer valuable guidance for those seeking to support their lymphatic health through the use of metal jewelry.

Chapter 18:
Choosing the Right Metal

Choosing the right metal for your individual needs is essential to maximize the benefits of metal therapy. Each metal has unique properties that can support various aspects of health and well-being. By personalizing metal therapy based on your specific health concerns and goals, you can enhance its effectiveness.

PERSONALIZING METAL THERAPY BASED ON INDIVIDUAL NEEDS
Identify Your Health Goals:

> Determine the specific health areas you want to focus on, such as immune support, hormonal balance, stress reduction, or skin health.

Understand Metal Properties:

> Familiarize yourself with the properties of different metals and their associated health benefits.

> - o Gold: Anti-inflammatory, hormonal balance, emotional stability.
> - o Silver: Antimicrobial, anti-inflammatory, skin health.
> - o Copper: Anti-inflammatory, pain relief, immune support.
> - o Platinum: Mental clarity, emotional stability, anti-aging.
> - o Titanium: Strength, durability, energy balance.

- o Cobalt: Hormonal regulation, tissue repair, immune support.
- o Stainless Steel: Hygiene, durability, general health.
- o Nickel: Muscle strength, joint health, nerve support.
- o Palladium: Hormonal regulation, antioxidant protection, stress response.

Assess Personal Health Needs:

Consider your current health conditions, sensitivities, and lifestyle. For example, if you have sensitive skin, hypoallergenic metals like platinum and stainless steel may be suitable.

Consult with Professionals:

Seek advice from healthcare professionals, holistic practitioners, or metal therapy experts to help you choose the right metal based on your individual health profile.

PRACTICAL TIPS FOR WEARING METAL JEWELRY
Start Gradually:

Begin by wearing one type of metal jewelry to observe how your body responds. Gradually introduce other metals as needed.

Choose the Right Type of Jewelry:

Select jewelry that aligns with your health goals. For instance, wear a gold ring for hormonal balance or a silver bracelet for skin health.

Rings: Ideal for targeting specific meridians and energy points.

Bracelets: Great for overall energy balance and immune support.

Necklaces: Beneficial for throat and chest-related concerns, such as respiratory health and emotional balance.

Earrings: Can influence head-related issues, including mental clarity and ear health.

Wear Jewelry Consistently:

Consistent use of metal jewelry allows for continuous exposure to the metal's beneficial properties. Wear the jewelry daily to maximize its effects.

Maintenance and Care:

Keep your metal jewelry clean and well-maintained to ensure its effectiveness and longevity. Use appropriate cleaning methods for each metal type.

Monitor Reactions:

Pay attention to how your body reacts to the metal. If you experience any irritation or discomfort, discontinue use and consult with a professional.

COMBINING METAL THERAPY WITH OTHER HOLISTIC PRACTICES
Energy Healing:

Integrate metal therapy with energy healing practices such as Reiki, acupuncture, or crystal therapy. Metals like gold and silver can enhance the flow of energy and amplify healing effects.

Meditation and Mindfulness:

> Use metal objects, such as gold-plated crystals or titanium beads, during meditation to enhance focus and promote a sense of calm. Wearing metal jewelry can also help ground your energy during mindfulness practices.

Aromatherapy:

> Combine metal therapy with aromatherapy by wearing metal jewelry infused with essential oils. Metals like copper and silver can enhance the absorption and benefits of the oils.

Diet and Nutrition:

> Support your metal therapy with a balanced diet rich in nutrients that complement the properties of the metals you are using. For example, consume foods high in antioxidants to enhance the anti-inflammatory effects of gold.

Physical Exercise:

> Wear metal jewelry during physical activities to support overall energy balance and enhance performance. Titanium jewelry is particularly beneficial for athletes due to its strength and durability.

Sleep and Relaxation:

> Incorporate metal therapy into your sleep routine by wearing metal jewelry that promotes relaxation and stress reduction. Gold and silver are excellent choices for enhancing sleep quality.

Choosing the right metal for your individual needs involves understanding the properties of different metals and aligning them with your health goals. By personalizing metal therapy, wearing metal jewelry consistently, and combining it with other holistic practices, you can enhance your overall health and well-being. Whether you seek to improve immune function, achieve hormonal balance, reduce stress, or support skin health, integrating metal therapy into your daily life offers a versatile and effective approach to achieving your wellness goals.

Metal Ring Meridian Balancing Technique

INTRODUCTION TO THE METAL RING MERIDIAN BALANCING TECHNIQUE

In holistic health practices, the concept of meridian balance plays a crucial role in maintaining overall well-being. The Metal Ring Meridian Balancing Technique leverages the use of specific metals and their placement on various fingers to enhance the body's natural energy flow and support different organ systems. This procedure is rooted in traditional practices such as Ayurveda and Traditional Chinese Medicine (TCM), where each finger is associated with different elements and meridians that influence various aspects of health.

UNDERSTANDING MERIDIANS

Meridians are channels through which life energy, or "Qi" (pronounced "chee"), flows in the body. These pathways connect different organs and systems, ensuring that energy circulates smoothly and efficiently. When meridians are balanced, the body functions optimally, but blockages or imbalances can lead to health issues. By targeting specific meridians through the placement of metal rings on corresponding fingers, this technique aims to restore balance and promote health.

HOW METALS AND MERIDIAN BALANCE WORK

Metals: Different metals are believed to possess unique properties that can influence the body's energy and physiological functions. For example, gold is thought to support circulatory health, while silver is renowned for its antimicrobial and immune-boosting properties. Wearing these metals on specific fingers can harness their potential benefits to balance and support various bodily systems.

Finger Placement: Each finger is associated with different elements, meridians, and organs in the body. By wearing a ring on a particular finger, the energy flow related to that finger can be influenced, enhancing the effectiveness of the metal's properties.

How to Muscle Test Using the O-Ring Method, the Arm Method, or the Body Method

Muscle testing, also known as applied kinesiology, is a technique used to assess the body's response to various stimuli by testing the strength of specific muscles. It can be used to determine the suitability of foods, supplements, or other substances for an individual. Here's a step-by-step guide on how to perform muscle testing using the O-Ring method, the Arm, and the Body method.

O-Ring Method
Step 1: Preparation

- Environment: Find a quiet, comfortable space free from distractions.
- State of Mind: Ensure you are calm and relaxed. Take a few deep breaths to center yourself.
- Hydration: Make sure you are well-hydrated, as dehydration can affect the results.

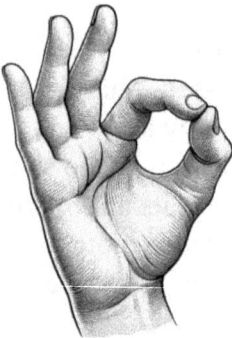

Step 2: Forming the O-Ring

• Hand Position: Use your dominant hand to form an "O" shape by touching the tip of your thumb to the tip of your index finger. This should create a small circle or ring.

- Baseline Test: Establish a baseline by asking a simple, truthful question such as "Is my name [your name]?" With your other hand, gently try to pull apart the O-Ring by inserting your thumb and index finger and applying a gentle outward force. Note the resistance. Your fingers should stay together, indicating a strong response.

Step 3: (INTENT)Testing a Substance or Question

- *Hold the Item*: If you are testing a substance, hold it in your free hand. If you are testing an abstract question, simply focus on the question.
- *Ask the Question:* Phrase your question clearly, for example, "Is this supplement beneficial for me?"
- *Apply Pressure*: With your other hand, try to pull apart the O-Ring again while focusing on your question or holding the substance.
- *Interpret the Result:*
  - Strong Response: If your fingers resist being pulled apart and the O-Ring stays intact, it indicates a positive response.
  - Weak Response: If your fingers easily pull apart, it indicates a negative response.

ARM METHOD
Step 1: Preparation

- Environment: Find a quiet, comfortable space free from distractions.
- State of Mind: Ensure you are calm and relaxed. Take a few deep breaths to center yourself.
- Hydration: Make sure you are well-hydrated, as dehydration can affect the results.

Step 2: Establishing a Baseline

- Position: Stand or sit comfortably. Extend one arm straight out in front of you, parallel to the ground.
- Baseline Test: Have a partner stand beside you. Ask a simple, truthful question such as "Is my name [your name]?" Your partner should gently press down on your extended arm just above the wrist while you resist the pressure. Note the strength of your resistance. Your arm should remain strong and resist the downward pressure.

Step 3: Testing a Substance or Question

- Hold the Item: If you are testing a substance, hold it in your free hand. If you are testing an abstract question, simply focus on the question.
- Ask the Question: Phrase your question clearly, for example, "Is this supplement beneficial for me?"
- Apply Pressure: Have your partner press down on your extended arm while you resist the pressure.
- Interpret the Result:
  - Strong Response: If your arm remains strong and resists the pressure, it indicates a positive response.
  - Weak Response: If your arm easily gives way to the pressure, it indicates a negative response.

BODY METHOD
Step 1: Preparation

- Environment: Find a quiet, comfortable space free from distractions.
- State of Mind: Ensure you are calm and relaxed. Take a few deep breaths to center yourself.

- Hydration: Make sure you are well-hydrated, as dehydration can affect the results.

Step 2: Establishing a Baseline

- Position: Stand comfortably.
- Program your subconscious mind and move forward for a "Yes" three times (3x). Then backward to program the "No" three times (3x)
- Baseline Test: Ask a simple, truthful question such as "Is my name [your name]?" Take a breath and relax. Let your body move freely. Forward is a "Yes," and backward is a "No."

Step 3: Testing a Substance or Question

- Hold the Item: If you are testing a substance, hold it in your free hand. If you are testing an abstract question, simply focus on the question.
- Ask the Question: Phrase your question clearly, for example, "Is this supplement beneficial for me?"
- Take a breath and relax. Let your body move freely. Forward is a "Yes," and backward is a "No."
- Interpret the Result:
  - Strong Response: If you move forward, it indicates a positive response.
  - Weak Response: If you move backward, it indicates a negative response.

Practical Tips

Consistency: Perform the tests under similar conditions each time to ensure consistency.

Record Results: Keep a journal of your findings, noting which substances or questions yield strong or weak responses.

Example Application

If you want to test whether a specific supplement is beneficial for you:

1. Establish Baseline: Using the O-Ring method, form an O-Ring and ask a simple, truthful question. Note the resistance.
2. Test the Supplement:
    a. Hold the supplement in your free hand.
    b. Ask, "Is this supplement beneficial for me?"
    c. Try to pull apart the O-Ring.
3. Interpret the Result:
    a. If the O-Ring stays intact (strong response), the supplement is likely beneficial.
    b. If the O-Ring pulls apart easily (weak response), the supplement may not be beneficial.

By following these steps, you can use muscle testing to gain insights into how different substances and questions affect your body.

***Practice using the O ring, arm, or body muscle testing until you acknowledge the baseline. If you are not familiar with muscle testing, this may take many days.

- Practice with saying your name, "Is my name __?__." You should be 100% accurate!
- Test another name, one that you have never been called.
- Keep practicing until you know your baseline!!!

Metal Ring Meridian Balancing Procedure: Step-by-Step Guide:

This procedure aims to identify which finger placement for a specific metal ring provides the strongest response in terms of balancing and supporting the body's systems.

1. Preparation (remove any other rings, including wedding ring before testing).
2. Establishing a Baseline
3. Intent: Think about your "Condition/Disease"
4. Choose a metal ring that corresponds to the system with a health condition you want to address (e.g., silver for respiratory health).
4. Hold or think about the "metal ring" and ask, *"Will wearing this __?__ metal ring balance __?__ body's condition?"*
5. Muscle Test Strength and Compare for the answer (using the "O ring" or "arm" or "body" test)
    a) If the answer is no, *choose another metal ring* and repeat the question.

    Sometimes, the "system" you think is the problem is not the main one causing the chaos. Trust your muscle-testing answer.

    b) *Muscle test, "Do I need more than one metal to balance __?__ my body's condition?"*
    c) Repeat with remaining metals.
5. Once you have determined a metal, now muscle test which finger(s) to wear the ring(s) on.
    - Little Finger: Place the metal ring on the little finger and test strength.
    - Ring Finger: Place the metal ring on the ring finger and test its strength.

- Middle Finger: Place the metal ring on the middle finger and test strength.
  - Index Finger: Place the metal ring on the index finger and test strength.
  - Thumb: Place the metal ring on the thumb and test strength.

For each finger, conduct the strength test and compare the results to find the strongest response.

Now, switch hands and repeat.

Determine the Strongest Response:

The finger that gives the strongest response is considered the most beneficial placement for wearing the metal ring to balance and support the specific organ system.

Benefits and Considerations

- Personalized Health Support: This procedure helps personalize the use of metal rings based on individual responses, potentially enhancing the effectiveness of traditional metal-based health practices.
- Non-Invasive: The method is non-invasive and can be easily performed at home with the help of a partner.
- Holistic Approach: Integrates traditional beliefs about metals and finger placements with modern muscle testing techniques to support overall health.

Additional Tips

- Consistency: Ensure consistent pressure is applied during each strength test to maintain accuracy.
- Multiple Trials: Conduct multiple trials for each finger to confirm the results and account for variability.

- Consultation: While this method can be a useful complementary practice, always consult with healthcare professionals for comprehensive health management.

The Organ Finger Correspondence procedure for constitutional organ balancing using metal rings is a practical method to determine the most beneficial finger placement for health support. By systematically testing and comparing strength responses, individuals can identify optimal ring placements to enhance their well-being.

TESTING FOR DURATION

Question Formulation: Phrase your questions clearly to determine the optimal duration. For example, "Is it beneficial for me to wear this ring for one hour?" Adjust the duration incrementally based on the responses.

1. Incremental Testing
   - 1 Hour: Hold the ring and ask, "Is it beneficial for me to wear this ring for one hour?" Perform the muscle test.
   - 2 Hours: If the response is strong for one hour, increase the duration incrementally. Ask, "Is it beneficial for me to wear this ring for two hours?" and perform the muscle test.
   - Continue Testing: Continue this process, increasing the duration incrementally (3 hours, 4 hours, etc.) until you identify the maximum duration that yields a strong response.
   - Maximum Daily Wear: Once you have identified the incremental durations, ask about the maximum daily wear. For example, "Is it beneficial for me to wear this ring for a total of 6 hours in one day?"
2. Validation and Adjustment

Monitor Results: Wear the ring for the tested duration and observe any physical, mental, or emotional changes. Adjust the duration based on your observations and subsequent muscle testing if necessary.

Example Application

If you tested a gold ring on your ring finger for anxiety:

- Establish Baseline: Using the O-Ring method, establish your baseline.

Test Duration:

- Ask, "Is it beneficial for me to wear this ring for one hour?" Perform the muscle test.
- If the response is strong, increase to two hours, and repeat.
- Continue until you find the maximum duration that yields a strong response.
- Maximum Daily Wear: Once you identify the duration, test for maximum daily wear. For example, "Is it beneficial for me to wear this ring for a total of 6 hours in one day?"
3. Regular Re-Evaluation: Re-evaluate the duration periodically to ensure it remains optimal as your condition changes.
4. WHEN TO STOP: Removal of the ring. Muscle test when to remove the ring. Mark it on your calendar! Do not over wear the metal ring!!!

*If you are allergic to any of the metals, DO NOT WEAR THEM!

Integrating Metal Therapy into Daily Life

Practical ways to integrate metal therapy into daily life, leveraging the benefits of various metals to support overall health and well-being. Metal therapy involves using metals such as gold, silver, copper, platinum, titanium, cobalt, stainless steel, and nickel in various forms to harness their healing properties.

The Concept of Metal Therapy

Metal therapy is rooted in ancient practices and has been used in various cultures to promote health, balance energy, and treat ailments. Each metal is believed to have unique properties that can influence physical, emotional, and spiritual health. Integrating metal therapy into daily life can be done through wearing jewelry, using metal-infused products, and incorporating metals into the environment.

Integrating Metal Therapy into Daily Life

Wearing Metal Jewelry:

Jewelry made from therapeutic metals can be worn to continuously benefit from their properties. Rings, bracelets, necklaces, and earrings made of specific metals can support targeted health benefits.

Using Metal-Infused Products:

Incorporate products infused with metals, such as creams, lotions, and hair care products. These products can deliver the benefits of metals directly to the skin and hair.

Metal Utensils and Cookware:

Using utensils and cookware made from beneficial metals like copper and stainless steel can ensure the purity of food and enhance its health benefits.

Home and Office Decor:

Decorate living and working spaces with metal objects. Items like metal sculptures, lamps, and furniture can contribute to a balanced and harmonious environment.

Energy Healing and Meditation:

Use metals in energy healing practices and meditation. Holding metal objects, such as crystals or metal beads, can enhance the flow of energy and support mental clarity and emotional balance.

Practical Tips for Daily Integration

Start with Jewelry:

Begin by wearing jewelry made from a metal that supports your specific health needs. For example, wear a silver bracelet for its antimicrobial properties or a gold ring for hormonal balance.

Incorporate Metal-Infused Products:

Choose skincare and haircare products that contain metal nanoparticles, like silver-infused creams or copper shampoos, to enhance your beauty routine with added health benefits.

Upgrade Your Kitchenware:

Invest in high-quality metal utensils and cookware. Copper pots and stainless steel utensils are excellent choices for both cooking and serving food.

Decorate with Intention:

Add metal elements to your home and office decor. Use brass candle holders, copper vases, or stainless steel sculptures to create a balanced and aesthetically pleasing environment.

Explore Energy Healing:

Experiment with metal tools in your meditation and energy healing practices. Use gold-plated crystals or hold a piece of titanium while meditating to amplify the healing effects.

Benefits of Integrating Metal Therapy

Physical Health:

Metals like silver and copper have antimicrobial properties that can support the immune system and skin health. Gold can help reduce inflammation and promote hormonal balance.

Emotional and Mental Well-being:

Wearing or using metals like platinum and titanium can enhance mental clarity, reduce stress, and promote emotional stability.

Energy Balance:

Metals can help balance the body's energy fields, promoting overall well-being and harmony. Gold and silver, for instance, are known for their conductive properties, which can enhance the flow of energy.

Enhanced Beauty and Aesthetics:

Metal-infused skincare and haircare products can improve the appearance of skin and hair, adding a touch of luxury to your daily routine.

Case Studies and Anecdotal Evidence

Case Study: Silver Jewelry for Skin Health:

> Background: A group of individuals with chronic skin conditions, such as eczema and psoriasis, wore silver bracelets daily for six months.

> Results: Participants reported significant improvements in skin condition, including reduced inflammation and fewer flare-ups. The antimicrobial properties of silver helped to soothe and protect the skin.

Case Study: Copper Cookware for Joint Health:

> Background: A study involving individuals with arthritis used copper cookware for all their meals over a period of one year.

> Results: Participants noted a reduction in joint pain and stiffness. The anti-inflammatory properties of copper, absorbed in trace amounts through food, contributed to the improvements.

Anecdotal Evidence: Gold Rings for Emotional Balance:

> Experience: Individuals wearing gold rings reported feeling more emotionally balanced and less stressed. The conductive properties of gold are believed to enhance the flow of energy and promote a sense of calm.

> Integrating metal therapy into daily life offers a holistic approach to enhancing physical, emotional, and spiritual health. By wearing metal jewelry, using metal-infused products, incorporating metal utensils and decor, and exploring energy healing practices, you can harness the unique properties of various metals to

support overall well-being. Whether through the antimicrobial effects of silver, the anti-inflammatory benefits of gold, or the mental clarity provided by platinum, metal therapy provides a versatile and effective means of promoting health and balance in everyday life.

Chapter 19:
Care and Maintenance of Metal Jewelry

Proper care and maintenance of metal jewelry are essential to ensure its longevity, aesthetic appeal, and continued efficacy in providing health benefits. Each metal requires specific cleaning and maintenance techniques to preserve its unique properties and prevent damage. Here's a comprehensive guide on how to care for different metals and maintain the efficacy of your metal jewelry.

How to Care for Different Metals

Gold:

> Cleaning: Clean gold jewelry with a solution of mild soap and warm water. Use a soft brush to gently scrub the jewelry, then rinse with clean water and pat dry with a soft cloth.

> Polishing: Use a gold polishing cloth to maintain its shine. Avoid abrasive cleaners that can scratch the surface.

> Storage: Store gold jewelry separately in a soft pouch or lined jewelry box to prevent scratches and tangling.

Silver:

Cleaning: Use a silver cleaning cloth or a solution of mild soap and water. For tarnish, use a silver polish or a homemade solution of baking soda and water.

Polishing: Regularly polish silver jewelry to prevent tarnish buildup. Avoid wearing silver in environments with high sulfur content to minimize tarnishing.

Storage: Store in an anti-tarnish cloth or a sealed plastic bag to reduce exposure to air and moisture.

Copper:

Cleaning: Clean copper jewelry with a mixture of lemon juice and salt or a solution of vinegar and salt. Rinse thoroughly and dry immediately to prevent corrosion.

Polishing: Use a copper polishing cloth to restore shine. Apply a thin layer of clear nail polish or wax to maintain its luster and prevent oxidation.

Storage: Store in a dry place and avoid exposure to moisture to prevent tarnish and corrosion.

Platinum:

Cleaning: Clean platinum jewelry with a solution of mild soap and warm water. Use a soft brush to gently scrub and then rinse thoroughly.

Polishing: Use a jewelry polishing cloth specifically designed for platinum to maintain its shine. Regular professional cleaning is recommended.

Storage: Store separately in a soft pouch or lined box to avoid scratches.

Titanium:

Cleaning: Clean titanium jewelry with mild soap and warm water. A soft cloth or brush can be used to remove dirt and grime.

Polishing: Use a titanium polishing cloth to maintain its shine. Avoid abrasive materials that can scratch the surface.

Storage: Store in a separate compartment to prevent scratches from harder metals.

Palladium:

Cleaning: Clean palladium jewelry with a mixture of mild soap and warm water. Use a soft cloth or a gentle brush to remove any dirt or grime. Rinse thoroughly with clean water and dry with a soft, lint-free cloth.

Polishing: Use a polishing cloth specifically designed for precious metals to maintain the appearance of palladium jewelry. Avoid using harsh chemicals or abrasive materials that can scratch or damage the surface.

Storage: Store palladium jewelry in a dry, cool place, preferably in a soft pouch or a jewelry box with a fabric lining. Keep it away from direct sunlight and moisture to prevent tarnishing and damage.

Cobalt:

Cleaning: Clean cobalt jewelry with mild soap and water. Rinse thoroughly and dry with a soft cloth.

Polishing: Use a polishing cloth for cobalt to maintain its appearance. Avoid harsh chemicals that can damage the surface.

Storage: Store in a dry, cool place away from direct sunlight and moisture.

Stainless Steel:

Cleaning: Clean stainless steel jewelry with a mixture of mild soap and warm water. Use a soft brush to remove dirt and debris.

Polishing: Use a stainless steel polishing cloth to maintain its shine. Stainless steel is resistant to tarnish, but regular cleaning keeps it looking new.

Storage: Store separately to prevent scratches, especially from harder metals.

Nickel:

Cleaning: Clean nickel jewelry with a mixture of mild soap and warm water. Use a soft cloth or brush to gently scrub away dirt and debris.

Deep Cleaning: For a deeper clean, soak the nickel item in the soap and water solution for a few minutes before scrubbing. Rinse thoroughly and dry with a soft cloth.

Polishing: Use a nickel polishing cloth to maintain its shine. Regular polishing helps keep the metal looking new and prevents the build-up of tarnish or grime.

Storage: Store nickel items separately from other metals to prevent scratches and contact that can lead to tarnish. Use individual pouches or soft cloth bags for each piece.

Avoid Moisture: Store nickel jewelry in a dry place. Excessive moisture can tarnish and degrade the appearance of the metal over time.

ENSURING THE LONGEVITY AND EFFICACY OF YOUR METAL JEWELRY

Regular Cleaning:

Clean your metal jewelry regularly to remove dirt, oils, and other residues that can accumulate and affect the metal's appearance and properties. Follow the specific cleaning guidelines for each metal.

Avoid Harsh Chemicals:

Avoid exposing your metal jewelry to harsh chemicals, such as chlorine, bleach, and household cleaners, which can damage the metal and cause discoloration. Remove jewelry before swimming or using cleaning products.

Proper Storage:

Store metal jewelry in a dry, cool place, away from direct sunlight and moisture. Use separate compartments, soft pouches, or lined jewelry boxes to prevent scratches and tangling.

Routine Inspection:

Regularly inspect your metal jewelry for signs of wear and tear, such as loose stones, scratches, or tarnish.

Address any issues promptly to prevent further damage.

Professional Maintenance:

Take your metal jewelry to a professional jeweler for regular maintenance and deep cleaning. Professional services can help restore the metal's shine and address any structural issues.

Avoid Impact:

Avoid wearing metal jewelry during activities that may cause impact or abrasion, such as sports or heavy manual work. This helps prevent scratches, dents, and other damage.

Temperature Considerations:

Be mindful of extreme temperatures, as they can affect certain metals. For example, rapid temperature changes can cause some metals to expand or contract, potentially leading to structural damage.

Use of Protective Coatings:

Apply protective coatings, such as clear nail polish or wax, to metals like copper and silver to prevent tarnish and oxidation. Reapply as needed to maintain protection.

Proper care and maintenance of metal jewelry are crucial for preserving its beauty, durability, and therapeutic properties. By following specific cleaning and storage guidelines for each metal, you can ensure the longevity and efficacy of your metal jewelry. Regular maintenance, professional inspections, and mindful usage will help keep your metal jewelry in excellent condition, allowing you to continue enjoying its benefits for years to come. Whether you wear gold for its anti-inflammatory properties or silver for its antimicrobial effects, maintaining your metal jewelry will enhance its role in supporting your overall health and well-being.

Chapter 20:
The Future of Metal-Based Therapies

Metal-based therapies have a rich history rooted in traditional medicine, and their future looks promising with emerging research and trends integrating traditional wisdom with modern science. This chapter explores the potential advancements in metal-based therapies and how combining ancient practices with contemporary scientific findings can enhance their efficacy and application.

Emerging Research and Trends

Nanotechnology and Metal Nanoparticles:

> Targeted Drug Delivery: Advances in nanotechnology are enabling the development of metal nanoparticles for targeted drug delivery. Metals like gold, silver, and platinum are being used to create nanoparticles that can deliver drugs directly to specific cells or tissues, increasing treatment efficacy and reducing side effects.

> Cancer Treatment: Gold nanoparticles are being explored for their potential in photothermal therapy, where they are used to target and destroy cancer cells with minimal damage to surrounding healthy tissues. This method shows promise in improving cancer treatment outcomes.

Antimicrobial Coatings:

> Medical Devices and Implants: Silver and copper are being used to create antimicrobial coatings for medical devices and implants. These coatings help prevent infections by inhibiting the growth of bacteria and other pathogens on the surfaces of medical equipment.

> Hospital Surfaces: Hospitals are adopting antimicrobial coatings for high-touch surfaces to reduce the risk of hospital-acquired infections. Silver-based coatings are particularly effective in maintaining sterile environments.

Metal-Based Supplements:

> Bioavailability Improvements: Research is focused on enhancing the bioavailability of metal-based supplements, such as zinc and magnesium, to improve their absorption and efficacy in the body. Advanced formulations aim to provide better health benefits with lower doses.

> Combination Therapies: Combining metal-based supplements with other nutrients and compounds is being studied to enhance their overall therapeutic effects. For example, combining copper with antioxidants to improve joint health and reduce inflammation.

Regenerative Medicine:

> Tissue Engineering: Metals like titanium and tantalum are being used in tissue engineering to create scaffolds that support the growth and regeneration of bone and soft tissues. These metal-based scaffolds are crucial in

developing advanced prosthetics and regenerative treatments.

Stem Cell Research: Research is exploring how metal ions and nanoparticles can influence stem cell differentiation and proliferation, potentially leading to breakthroughs in regenerative medicine and tissue repair.

Personalized Medicine:

Customized Therapies: Advances in genomics and biotechnology are paving the way for personalized metal-based therapies tailored to an individual's genetic profile and specific health needs. This approach aims to maximize therapeutic benefits while minimizing risks and side effects.

Wearable Technology: Integrating metal-based materials into wearable health monitoring devices can provide real-time data on an individual's health status, enabling personalized treatment plans and early intervention for various conditions.

Integrating Traditional Wisdom with Modern Science

Reevaluating Traditional Practices:

Evidence-Based Validation: Modern research is increasingly validating the efficacy of traditional metal-based therapies. Studies are investigating the mechanisms behind the health benefits of metals like gold, silver, and copper, providing scientific backing to age-old practices.

Holistic Approaches: Integrating traditional wisdom with modern medical practices offers a holistic approach to health. This integration considers not only physical but also emotional and spiritual well-being, aligning with the principles of holistic medicine.

Combining Modalities:

Complementary Therapies: Combining metal-based therapies with other complementary therapies, such as acupuncture, herbal medicine, and aromatherapy, can enhance overall treatment outcomes. For example, using gold acupuncture needles in conjunction with traditional herbal remedies for hormonal balance.

Integrative Health Programs: Developing integrative health programs that include metal-based therapies alongside conventional treatments can provide comprehensive care. These programs can be tailored to address specific conditions, such as chronic pain, autoimmune disorders, and mental health issues.

Cultural Sensitivity and Accessibility:

Respecting Cultural Practices: Recognizing and respecting the cultural significance of traditional metal-based therapies is essential. Integrating these practices into modern healthcare systems can make treatments more accessible and acceptable to diverse populations.

Education and Awareness: Promoting education and awareness about the benefits of metal-based therapies can help bridge the gap between traditional and modern medicine. Healthcare providers and patients can benefit from understanding how these therapies can complement conventional treatments.

Sustainable and Ethical Practices:

> Sustainable Sourcing: Ensuring the sustainable and ethical sourcing of metals used in therapies is crucial. This includes responsible mining practices and the recycling of metals to minimize environmental impact.

> Ethical Research: Conducting ethical research and clinical trials on metal-based therapies ensures that treatments are safe, effective, and beneficial for patients. Transparency in research practices and results is essential for maintaining trust and credibility.

The future of metal-based therapies lies in the seamless integration of traditional wisdom with modern scientific advancements. Emerging research and trends in nanotechnology, antimicrobial coatings, regenerative medicine, and personalized treatments are poised to enhance the efficacy and application of metal-based therapies. By combining ancient practices with contemporary findings, we can create holistic, effective, and sustainable approaches to health and well-being. As research continues to evolve, metal-based therapies will likely play an increasingly significant role in modern healthcare, offering innovative solutions for a wide range of health conditions.

Chapter 21:
By Health Conditions

In holistic health practices, the use of specific metals is believed to balance various bodily systems and support overall well-being. This section explores a selection of common diseases and conditions, the metals traditionally used to balance the affected systems, and the recommended finger placement for wearing rings made of these metals. The practice of wearing metal rings on specific fingers is rooted in ancient traditions such as Ayurveda and Traditional Chinese Medicine (TCM), which associate each finger with different elements and meridians that influence various aspects of health.

Top Ten Common Conditions starting with "A"

1. Asthma

- System of the Body: Respiratory System
- Metal to Balance: Silver (for respiratory health)
- Ring Finger Placement: Little Finger — associated with the heart and small intestine meridians, influencing lung health.

2. Anemia

- System of the Body: Circulatory System
- Metal to Balance: Copper (supports red blood cell formation)
- Ring Finger Placement: Middle Finger – associated with blood circulation and supporting overall vitality.

3. Arthritis

- System of the Body: Musculoskeletal System
- Metal to Balance: Copper (reduces inflammation and supports joint health)
- Ring Finger Placement: Index Finger – influences the meridian associated with joint health.

4. Alzheimer's Disease

- System of the Body: Nervous System
- Metal to Balance: Platinum (supports brain health and mental clarity)
- Ring Finger Placement: Thumb – linked to the brain and cognitive function.

5. Anxiety

- System of the Body: Nervous System
- Metal to Balance: Silver (calms and soothes the mind)
- Ring Finger Placement: Middle Finger – supports mental health and reduces stress.

6. Acne

- System of the Body: Integumentary System (Skin)
- Metal to Balance: Silver (antimicrobial and anti-inflammatory)
- Ring Finger Placement: Ring Finger – influences skin health and clarity.

7. Allergies

- System of the Body: Immune System
- Metal to Balance: Stainless Steel (supports immune function and reduces inflammation)
- Ring Finger Placement: Index Finger – helps balance immune response.

8. Anorexia Nervosa

- System of the Body: Digestive System
- Metal to Balance: Copper (supports digestion and nutrient absorption)
- Ring Finger Placement: Middle Finger – influences digestive health and metabolism.

9 Arrhythmia

- System of the Body: Circulatory System
- Metal to Balance: Gold (supports heart health and stabilizes heart rhythm)
- Ring Finger Placement: Ring Finger – crucial for the heart's electrical conduction system.

10. Ankylosing Spondylitis

- System of the Body: Musculoskeletal System
- Metal to Balance: Titanium (supports bone health and reduces inflammation)
- Ring Finger Placement: Index Finger – associated with the spine and joint health.

Top Ten Common Conditions starting with "B"

1. Bronchitis

- System of the Body: Respiratory System
- Metal to Balance: Silver (calms and reduces inflammation)
- Ring Finger Placement: Little Finger – supports lung health and reduces respiratory inflammation.

2. Bacterial Infections

- System of the Body: Immune System
- Metal to Balance: Silver (antimicrobial properties)
- Ring Finger Placement: Index Finger – enhances immune function to combat infections.

3. Bipolar Disorder

- System of the Body: Nervous System
- Metal to Balance: Platinum (stabilizes mood and supports mental clarity)
- Ring Finger Placement: Thumb – influences brain and cognitive function.

4. Bladder Infections (Cystitis)

- System of the Body: Urinary System
- Metal to Balance: Cobalt (supports urinary health and reduces inflammation)
- Ring Finger Placement: Index Finger – linked to bladder and urinary tract health.

5. Blood Pressure (High)

- System of the Body: Circulatory System
- Metal to Balance: Silver (calms and reduces stress)
- Ring Finger Placement: Index Finger – influences meridian associated with blood pressure regulation.

6. Blood Pressure (Low)

- System of the Body: Circulatory System
- Metal to Balance: Gold (energizes and strengthens)
- Ring Finger Placement: Ring Finger – enhances heart function and energy flow.

7. Bone Fractures

- System of the Body: Skeletal System
- Metal to Balance: Titanium (supports bone health and healing)
- Ring Finger Placement: Middle Finger – aids in bone repair and structural integrity.

8. Bronchial Asthma

- System of the Body: Respiratory System
- Metal to Balance: Silver (supports respiratory function and reduces inflammation)
- Ring Finger Placement: Little Finger – associated with lung health and function.

9. Breast Cancer

- System of the Body: Immune System
- Metal to Balance: Gold (supports immune function and vitality)
- Ring Finger Placement: Thumb – supports immune response and overall health.

10. Bursitis

- System of the Body: Musculoskeletal System
- Metal to Balance: Copper (reduces inflammation and supports joint health)
- Ring Finger Placement: Index Finger – supports joint and muscle health.

Top Ten Common Conditions starting with "C"

1. Cancer

- System of the Body: Various (depends on type, e.g., immune system, circulatory system)
- Metal to Balance: Platinum (supports overall health and cell function)
- Ring Finger Placement: Thumb – influences general vitality and immune support.

2. Cardiomyopathy

- System of the Body: Circulatory System
- Metal to Balance: Gold (enhances heart muscle strength)
- Ring Finger Placement: Ring Finger – strengthens and supports the heart meridian.

3. Cataracts

- System of the Body: Sensory System (Eyes)
- Metal to Balance: Silver (calms and supports eye health)
- Ring Finger Placement: Index Finger – linked to vision and eye health.

4. Chronic Fatigue Syndrome (CFS)

- System of the Body: Nervous System
- Metal to Balance: Gold (energizes and supports overall vitality)
- Ring Finger Placement: Ring Finger – enhances energy levels and supports cardiovascular health.

5. Cirrhosis

- System of the Body: Digestive System (Liver)
- Metal to Balance: Copper (supports liver function and detoxification)
- Ring Finger Placement: Middle Finger – aids in liver health and metabolic balance.

6. Colitis

- System of the Body: Digestive System (Colon)
- Metal to Balance: Copper (reduces inflammation and supports digestive health)
- Ring Finger Placement: Index Finger – supports intestinal health and reduces inflammation.

7. Common Cold

- System of the Body: Immune System
- Metal to Balance: Silver (antimicrobial and supports immune function)
- Ring Finger Placement: Index Finger – enhances immune response and respiratory health.

8. Congestive Heart Failure (CHF)

- System of the Body: Circulatory System
- Metal to Balance: Gold (strengthens and supports heart function)
- Ring Finger Placement: Ring Finger – associated with the heart meridian, enhancing cardiac strength.

9. Constipation

- System of the Body: Digestive System
- Metal to Balance: Copper (supports digestive health and bowel movement)
- Ring Finger Placement: Middle Finger – influences digestive health and promotes regularity.

10. Crohn's Disease

- System of the Body: Digestive System
- Metal to Balance: Copper (reduces inflammation and supports intestinal health)
- Ring Finger Placement: Index Finger – supports digestive health and reduces gastrointestinal inflammation.

Top Ten Common Conditions starting with "D"

1. Depression

- System of the Body: Nervous System
- Metal to Balance: Platinum (supports mental clarity and emotional balance)
- Ring Finger Placement: Thumb – influences brain function and mental health.

2. Diabetes

- System of the Body: Endocrine System
- Metal to Balance: Copper (supports metabolic processes and blood sugar regulation)
- Ring Finger Placement: Middle Finger – supports metabolic health and endocrine balance.

3. Dermatitis

- System of the Body: Integumentary System (Skin)
- Metal to Balance: Silver (antimicrobial and anti-inflammatory)
- Ring Finger Placement: Ring Finger – supports skin health and reduces inflammation.

4. Diarrhea

- System of the Body: Digestive System
- Metal to Balance: Copper (supports digestive health and reduces inflammation)
- Ring Finger Placement: Middle Finger – influences digestive health and promotes balance.

5. Diverticulitis

- System of the Body: Digestive System
- Metal to Balance: Copper (reduces inflammation and supports intestinal health)
- Ring Finger Placement: Index Finger – supports intestinal health and reduces inflammation.

6. Dizziness

- System of the Body: Nervous System
- Metal to Balance: Platinum (stabilizes and supports brain function)
- Ring Finger Placement: Thumb – influences balance and brain function.

7. Dysmenorrhea

- System of the Body: Reproductive System
- Metal to Balance: Gold (supports reproductive health and reduces pain)
- Ring Finger Placement: Ring Finger – enhances reproductive health and reduces menstrual discomfort.

8. Dyspnea (Shortness of Breath)

- System of the Body: Respiratory System
- Metal to Balance: Silver (supports respiratory function and reduces inflammation)
- Ring Finger Placement: Little Finger – influences lung health and respiratory function.

9. Dysphagia (Difficulty Swallowing)

- System of the Body: Digestive System
- Metal to Balance: Copper (supports digestive health and esophageal function)
- Ring Finger Placement: Index Finger – supports esophageal and digestive health.

10. Dystonia

- System of the Body: Nervous System
- Metal to Balance: Platinum (supports neurological function and reduces muscle contractions)
- Ring Finger Placement: Thumb – influences muscle and nerve function.

Top Ten Common Conditions starting with "E"

1. Eczema

- System of the Body: Integumentary System (Skin)
- Metal to Balance: Silver (anti-inflammatory and antimicrobial)
- Ring Finger Placement: Ring Finger – supports skin health and reduces inflammation.

2. Edema

- System of the Body: Circulatory System
- Metal to Balance: Copper (supports fluid balance and reduces swelling)
- Ring Finger Placement: Little Finger – aids in reducing fluid retention and improving circulation.

3. Emphysema

- System of the Body: Respiratory System
- Metal to Balance: Silver (supports respiratory function and reduces inflammation)
- Ring Finger Placement: Little Finger – enhances lung health and respiratory function.

4. Endocarditis

- System of the Body: Circulatory System
- Metal to Balance: Silver (antimicrobial and anti-inflammatory)
- Ring Finger Placement: Middle Finger – helps reduce inflammation and supports heart health.

5. Endometriosis

- System of the Body: Reproductive System
- Metal to Balance: Gold (supports reproductive health and reduces pain)
- Ring Finger Placement: Ring Finger – enhances reproductive health and reduces menstrual discomfort.

6. Epilepsy

- System of the Body: Nervous System
- Metal to Balance: Platinum (supports neurological function and reduces seizures)
- Ring Finger Placement: Thumb – influences brain function and supports neural health.

7. Erectile Dysfunction

- System of the Body: Reproductive System
- Metal to Balance: Gold (enhances reproductive health and vitality)
- Ring Finger Placement: Ring Finger – supports reproductive health and vitality.

8. Esophagitis

- System of the Body: Digestive System (Esophagus)
- Metal to Balance: Copper (reduces inflammation and supports esophageal health)
- Ring Finger Placement: Index Finger – aids in esophageal and digestive health.

9. Essential Tremor

- System of the Body: Nervous System
- Metal to Balance: Platinum (stabilizes and supports brain function)
- Ring Finger Placement: Thumb – influences motor control and brain function.

10. Eye Strain

- System of the Body: Sensory System (Eyes)
- Metal to Balance: Silver (calms and supports eye health)
- Ring Finger Placement: Index Finger – linked to vision and eye health.

Top Ten Common Conditions starting with "F"

1. Fatigue

- System of the Body: Nervous System
- Metal to Balance: Gold (energizes and supports overall vitality)
- Ring Finger Placement: Ring Finger – enhances energy levels and supports general vitality.

2. Fibromyalgia

- System of the Body: Musculoskeletal System
- Metal to Balance: Copper (reduces inflammation and supports muscle health)
- Ring Finger Placement: Middle Finger – aids in reducing pain and supporting muscle function.

3. Flu (Influenza)

- System of the Body: Immune System
- Metal to Balance: Silver (antimicrobial and supports immune function)
- Ring Finger Placement: Index Finger – enhances immune response and respiratory health.

4. Fractures

- System of the Body: Skeletal System
- Metal to Balance: Titanium (supports bone healing and strength)
- Ring Finger Placement: Middle Finger – aids in bone repair and structural integrity.

5. Fungal Infections

- System of the Body: Integumentary System (Skin)
- Metal to Balance: Silver (antimicrobial and antifungal)
- Ring Finger Placement: Ring Finger – supports skin health and reduces infection.

6. Frozen Shoulder

- System of the Body: Musculoskeletal System
- Metal to Balance: Copper (reduces inflammation and supports joint health)
- Ring Finger Placement: Index Finger – supports joint mobility and reduces inflammation.

7. Fibroids

- System of the Body: Reproductive System
- Metal to Balance: Gold (supports reproductive health and reduces growth)
- Ring Finger Placement: Ring Finger – enhances reproductive health and reduces discomfort.

8. Flatulence

- System of the Body: Digestive System
- Metal to Balance: Copper (supports digestive health and reduces gas)
- Ring Finger Placement: Middle Finger – aids in digestive function and reduces bloating.

9. Folliculitis

- System of the Body: Integumentary System (Skin)
- Metal to Balance: Silver (antimicrobial and anti-inflammatory)
- Ring Finger Placement: Ring Finger – supports skin health and reduces infection.

10. Food Poisoning

- System of the Body: Digestive System
- Metal to Balance: Copper (supports detoxification and digestive health)
- Ring Finger Placement: Middle Finger – aids in digestive recovery and reduces inflammation.

Top Ten Common Conditions starting with "G"

1. Gallstones

- System of the Body: Digestive System (Gallbladder)
- Metal to Balance: Copper (supports liver and gallbladder function)
- Ring Finger Placement: Middle Finger – aids in gallbladder health and digestive function.

2. Gastritis

- System of the Body: Digestive System (Stomach)
- Metal to Balance: Copper (reduces inflammation and supports stomach health)
- Ring Finger Placement: Middle Finger – supports digestive health and reduces gastric inflammation.

3. Gastroenteritis

- System of the Body: Digestive System
- Metal to Balance: Copper (supports digestive health and reduces inflammation)
- Ring Finger Placement: Middle Finger – aids in digestive recovery and reduces inflammation.

4. Gastroesophageal Reflux Disease (GERD)

- System of the Body: Digestive System (Esophagus)
- Metal to Balance: Copper (supports esophageal health and reduces acid)
- Ring Finger Placement: Index Finger – aids in esophageal and digestive health.

5. Glaucoma

- System of the Body: Sensory System (Eyes)
- Metal to Balance: Silver (calms and supports eye health)
- Ring Finger Placement: Index Finger – linked to vision and eye health.

6. Gout

- System of the Body: Musculoskeletal System
- Metal to Balance: Copper (reduces inflammation and supports joint health)
- Ring Finger Placement: Index Finger – supports joint health and reduces inflammation.

7. Graves' Disease

- System of the Body: Endocrine System (Thyroid)
- Metal to Balance: Copper (supports thyroid function and reduces inflammation)
- Ring Finger Placement: Middle Finger – supports endocrine health and thyroid balance.

8. Guillain-Barré Syndrome

- System of the Body: Nervous System
- Metal to Balance: Platinum (supports neurological function and recovery)
- Ring Finger Placement: Thumb – influences nerve function and supports recovery.

9. Gum Disease (Periodontitis)

- System of the Body: Oral Health (Gums)
- Metal to Balance: Silver (antimicrobial and supports oral health)
- Ring Finger Placement: Index Finger – supports gum health and reduces inflammation.

10. Gynecomastia

- System of the Body: Endocrine System
- Metal to Balance: Gold (supports hormonal balance)
- Ring Finger Placement: Ring Finger – aids in hormonal balance and endocrine health.

Top Ten Common Conditions starting with "H"

1. Hair Loss (Alopecia)

- System of the Body: Integumentary System (Scalp/Hair)
- Metal to Balance: Copper (supports hair health and growth)
- Ring Finger Placement: Ring Finger – enhances scalp and hair health.

2. Halitosis (Bad Breath)

- System of the Body: Oral Health
- Metal to Balance: Silver (antimicrobial and supports oral health)
- Ring Finger Placement: Index Finger – supports oral health and reduces bacterial growth.

3. Hay Fever (Allergic Rhinitis)

- System of the Body: Immune System
- Metal to Balance: Stainless Steel (supports immune function and reduces inflammation)
- Ring Finger Placement: Index Finger – enhances immune response and reduces allergy symptoms.

4. Headache

- System of the Body: Nervous System
- Metal to Balance: Platinum (supports neurological function and reduces pain)
- Ring Finger Placement: Thumb – influences brain function and reduces headache symptoms.

5. Hearing Loss

- System of the Body: Sensory System (Ears)
- Metal to Balance: Silver (supports auditory health)
- Ring Finger Placement: Index Finger – enhances auditory function and ear health.

6. Heart Disease

- System of the Body: Circulatory System
- Metal to Balance: Gold (supports heart health and function)
- Ring Finger Placement: Ring Finger – enhances cardiovascular health and supports heart function.

7. Hemorrhoids

- System of the Body: Digestive System (Rectum/Anus)
- Metal to Balance: Copper (reduces inflammation and supports digestive health)
- Ring Finger Placement: Middle Finger – supports digestive health and reduces inflammation.

8. Hepatitis

- System of the Body: Digestive System (Liver)
- Metal to Balance: Copper (supports liver health and reduces inflammation)
- Ring Finger Placement: Middle Finger – enhances liver function and supports detoxification.

9. Herpes

- System of the Body: Immune System
- Metal to Balance: Silver (antimicrobial and supports immune function)
- Ring Finger Placement: Index Finger – supports immune response and reduces viral activity.

10. Hypertension (High Blood Pressure)

- System of the Body: Circulatory System
- Metal to Balance: Silver (calms and reduces stress)
- Ring Finger Placement: Index Finger – influences meridian associated with blood pressure regulation.

Top Ten Common Conditions starting with "I"

1. IBS (Irritable Bowel Syndrome)

- System of the Body: Digestive System
- Metal to Balance: Copper (supports digestive health and reduces inflammation)
- Ring Finger Placement: Middle Finger – enhances digestive function and reduces symptoms.

2. Impetigo

- System of the Body: Integumentary System (Skin)
- Metal to Balance: Silver (antimicrobial and supports skin health)
- Ring Finger Placement: Ring Finger – supports skin health and reduces infection.

3. Incontinence

- System of the Body: Urinary System
- Metal to Balance: Cobalt (supports urinary health and reduces inflammation)
- Ring Finger Placement: Index Finger – supports bladder health and reduces symptoms.

4. Indigestion

- System of the Body: Digestive System
- Metal to Balance: Copper (supports digestive health and reduces discomfort)
- Ring Finger Placement: Middle Finger – enhances digestive function and reduces symptoms.

5. Infertility

- System of the Body: Reproductive System
- Metal to Balance: Gold (supports reproductive health and vitality)
- Ring Finger Placement: Ring Finger – enhances reproductive health and supports fertility.

6. Influenza (Flu)

- System of the Body: Immune System
- Metal to Balance: Silver (antimicrobial and supports immune function)
- Ring Finger Placement: Index Finger – enhances immune response and respiratory health.

7. Ingrown Toenail

- System of the Body: Integumentary System (Nails)
- Metal to Balance: Silver (antimicrobial and reduces inflammation)
- Ring Finger Placement: Ring Finger – supports nail health and reduces infection.

8. Insomnia

- System of the Body: Nervous System
- Metal to Balance: Platinum (calms and supports sleep)
- Ring Finger Placement: Thumb – enhances mental calmness and supports restful sleep.

9. Iron Deficiency Anemia

- System of the Body: Circulatory System
- Metal to Balance: Copper (supports red blood cell production)
- Ring Finger Placement: Middle Finger – enhances blood health and supports iron absorption.

10. Ischemia

- System of the Body: Circulatory System
- Metal to Balance: Gold (supports heart health and improves circulation)
- Ring Finger Placement: Ring Finger – enhances cardiovascular function and improves blood flow.

Top Ten Common Conditions starting with "J"

1. Jaundice

- System of the Body: Digestive System (Liver)
- Metal to Balance: Copper (supports liver health and reduces bilirubin levels)
- Ring Finger Placement: Middle Finger – enhances liver function and supports detoxification.

2. Jaw Pain (TMJ Disorder)

- System of the Body: Musculoskeletal System (Jaw)
- Metal to Balance: Copper (reduces inflammation and supports joint health)
- Ring Finger Placement: Index Finger – supports joint health and reduces inflammation.

3. Joint Pain (Arthralgia)

- System of the Body: Musculoskeletal System
- Metal to Balance: Copper (reduces inflammation and supports joint health)
- Ring Finger Placement: Index Finger – supports joint health and reduces pain.

4. Juvenile Diabetes (Type 1 Diabetes)

- System of the Body: Endocrine System (Pancreas)
- Metal to Balance: Copper (supports metabolic processes and blood sugar regulation)
- Ring Finger Placement: Middle Finger – supports endocrine health and blood sugar balance.

5. Jock Itch (Tinea Cruris)

- System of the Body: Integumentary System (Skin)
- Metal to Balance: Silver (antimicrobial and antifungal)
- Ring Finger Placement: Ring Finger – supports skin health and reduces fungal infection.

6. Joint Effusion (Fluid in the Joint)

- System of the Body: Musculoskeletal System
- Metal to Balance: Copper (reduces inflammation and supports joint health)
- Ring Finger Placement: Index Finger – supports joint health and reduces fluid accumulation.

7. Jet Lag

- System of the Body: Nervous System
- Metal to Balance: Platinum (supports mental clarity and regulates sleep cycles)
- Ring Finger Placement: Thumb – enhances brain function and supports sleep regulation.

8. Juvenile Rheumatoid Arthritis (JRA)

- System of the Body: Musculoskeletal System
- Metal to Balance: Copper (reduces inflammation and supports joint health)
- Ring Finger Placement: Index Finger – supports joint health and reduces inflammation.

9. Jaw Fracture

- System of the Body: Musculoskeletal System (Jaw)
- Metal to Balance: Titanium (supports bone healing and strength)
- Ring Finger Placement: Middle Finger – aids in bone repair and structural integrity.

10. Jejunitis

- System of the Body: Digestive System (Small Intestine)
- Metal to Balance: Copper (supports digestive health and reduces inflammation)
- Ring Finger Placement: Middle Finger – enhances intestinal health and supports digestion.

Top Ten Common Conditions starting with "K"

1. Kidney Stones

- System of the Body: Urinary System
- Metal to Balance: Cobalt (supports urinary health and reduces stone formation)
- Ring Finger Placement: Index Finger – supports kidney function and urinary health.

2. Keratitis

- System of the Body: Sensory System (Eyes)
- Metal to Balance: Silver (antimicrobial and supports eye health)
- Ring Finger Placement: Index Finger – enhances eye health and reduces infection.

3. Keratosis Pilaris

- System of the Body: Integumentary System (Skin)
- Metal to Balance: Silver (supports skin health and reduces inflammation)
- Ring Finger Placement: Ring Finger – supports skin health and reduces keratin buildup.

4. Klinefelter Syndrome

- System of the Body: Endocrine System
- Metal to Balance: Gold (supports hormonal balance and overall health)
- Ring Finger Placement: Ring Finger – enhances endocrine function and supports hormonal health.

5. Kyphosis

- System of the Body: Musculoskeletal System (Spine)
- Metal to Balance: Titanium (supports spinal health and structural integrity)
- Ring Finger Placement: Middle Finger – supports spine health and alignment.

6. Kawasaki Disease

- System of the Body: Circulatory System
- Metal to Balance: Gold (supports heart health and reduces inflammation)
- Ring Finger Placement: Ring Finger – enhances cardiovascular health and reduces inflammation.

7. Keratoconus

- System of the Body: Sensory System (Eyes)
- Metal to Balance: Silver (supports corneal health)
- Ring Finger Placement: Index Finger – enhances eye health and supports corneal stability.

8. Knee Pain

- System of the Body: Musculoskeletal System (Knee)
- Metal to Balance: Copper (reduces inflammation and supports joint health)
- Ring Finger Placement: Index Finger – supports knee joint health and reduces pain.

9. Kidney Infection (Pyelonephritis)

- System of the Body: Urinary System
- Metal to Balance: Cobalt (supports kidney health and reduces infection)
- Ring Finger Placement: Index Finger – supports kidney function and reduces inflammation.

10. Keratoderma (Palmoplantar Keratoderma)

- System of the Body: Integumentary System (Skin)
- Metal to Balance: Silver (supports skin health and reduces thickening)
- Ring Finger Placement: Ring Finger – supports skin health and reduces keratin buildup.

Top Ten Common Conditions starting with "L"

1. Laryngitis

- System of the Body: Respiratory System
- Metal to Balance: Silver (calms and reduces inflammation)
- Ring Finger Placement: Little Finger – supports throat health and reduces inflammation.

2. Leukemia

- System of the Body: Circulatory System
- Metal to Balance: Silver (supports immune function and reduces inflammation)
- Ring Finger Placement: Thumb – influences bone marrow and blood cell production.

3. Liver Disease

- System of the Body: Digestive System (Liver)
- Metal to Balance: Copper (supports liver health and detoxification)
- Ring Finger Placement: Middle Finger – enhances liver function and supports detoxification.

4. Lupus

- System of the Body: Immune System
- Metal to Balance: Silver (reduces inflammation and supports immune function)
- Ring Finger Placement: Index Finger – enhances immune response and reduces autoimmune symptoms.

5. Lyme Disease

- System of the Body: Immune System
- Metal to Balance: Silver (antimicrobial and supports immune function)
- Ring Finger Placement: Index Finger – supports immune response and reduces bacterial infection.

6. Lymphedema

- System of the Body: Lymphatic System
- Metal to Balance: Copper (supports lymphatic drainage and reduces swelling)
- Ring Finger Placement: Little Finger – supports lymphatic health and reduces fluid retention.

7. Lymphoma

- System of the Body: Immune System (Lymphatic System)
- Metal to Balance: Silver (supports immune function and reduces inflammation)
- Ring Finger Placement: Index Finger – enhances immune response and supports lymphatic health.

8. Low Blood Pressure (Hypotension)

- System of the Body: Circulatory System
- Metal to Balance: Gold (energizes and strengthens)
- Ring Finger Placement: Ring Finger – enhances heart function and energy flow.

9. Lactose Intolerance

- System of the Body: Digestive System
- Metal to Balance: Copper (supports digestive enzymes and reduces discomfort)
- Ring Finger Placement: Middle Finger – aids in digestive function and reduces symptoms.

10. Lichen Planus

- System of the Body: Integumentary System (Skin)
- Metal to Balance: Silver (antimicrobial and supports skin health)
- Ring Finger Placement: Ring Finger – supports skin health and reduces inflammation.

Top Ten Common Conditions starting with "M"

1. Malaria

- System of the Body: Immune System
- Metal to Balance: Silver (antimicrobial and supports immune function)
- Ring Finger Placement: Index Finger – enhances immune response and reduces parasitic infection.

2. Meniere's Disease

- System of the Body: Sensory System (Ears)
- Metal to Balance: Silver (supports ear health and reduces inflammation)
- Ring Finger Placement: Index Finger – supports auditory function and reduces vertigo symptoms.

3. Menopause Symptoms

- System of the Body: Endocrine System
- Metal to Balance: Gold (supports hormonal balance)
- Ring Finger Placement: Ring Finger – enhances endocrine function and reduces menopausal symptoms.

4. Migraine

- System of the Body: Nervous System
- Metal to Balance: Platinum (supports neurological function and reduces pain)
- Ring Finger Placement: Thumb – influences brain function and reduces migraine symptoms.

5. Mitral Valve Prolapse

- System of the Body: Circulatory System (Heart)
- Metal to Balance: Gold (supports heart health and function)
- Ring Finger Placement: Ring Finger – enhances cardiovascular health and supports heart function.

6. Mononucleosis

- System of the Body: Immune System
- Metal to Balance: Silver (supports immune function and reduces viral activity)
- Ring Finger Placement: Index Finger – enhances immune response and reduces infection.

7. Multiple Sclerosis (MS)

- System of the Body: Nervous System
- Metal to Balance: Platinum (supports neurological function and reduces symptoms)
- Ring Finger Placement: Thumb – enhances brain function and supports nerve health.

8. Muscle Cramps

- System of the Body: Muscular System
- Metal to Balance: Copper (reduces inflammation and supports muscle health)
- Ring Finger Placement: Index Finger – supports muscle health and reduces cramps.

9. Myasthenia Gravis

- System of the Body: Nervous System
- Metal to Balance: Platinum (supports neurological function and reduces muscle weakness)
- Ring Finger Placement: Thumb – influences nerve function and supports muscle strength.

10. Myocardial Infarction (Heart Attack)

- System of the Body: Circulatory System (Heart)
- Metal to Balance: Gold (supports heart health and recovery)
- Ring Finger Placement: Ring Finger – enhances cardiovascular health and supports heart function.

Top Ten Common Conditions starting with "N"

1. Narcolepsy

- System of the Body: Nervous System
- Metal to Balance: Platinum (supports neurological function and regulates sleep)
- Ring Finger Placement: Thumb – enhances brain function and supports sleep regulation.

2. Nasal Polyps

- System of the Body: Respiratory System
- Metal to Balance: Silver (reduces inflammation and supports respiratory health)
- Ring Finger Placement: Little Finger – supports nasal passage health and reduces inflammation.

3. Nausea

- System of the Body: Digestive System
- Metal to Balance: Copper (supports digestive health and reduces discomfort)
- Ring Finger Placement: Middle Finger – aids in digestive function and reduces symptoms.

4. Nephritis

- System of the Body: Urinary System (Kidneys)
- Metal to Balance: Cobalt (supports kidney health and reduces inflammation)
- Ring Finger Placement: Index Finger – supports kidney function and reduces inflammation.

5. Neuralgia

- System of the Body: Nervous System
- Metal to Balance: Platinum (supports nerve health and reduces pain)
- Ring Finger Placement: Thumb – influences nerve function and reduces pain.

6. Neuritis

- System of the Body: Nervous System
- Metal to Balance: Platinum (supports nerve health and reduces inflammation)
- Ring Finger Placement: Thumb – enhances nerve function and reduces symptoms.

7. Neuropathy

- System of the Body: Nervous System
- Metal to Balance: Platinum (supports neurological function and reduces symptoms)
- Ring Finger Placement: Thumb – influences nerve function and supports nerve health.

8. Night Blindness

- System of the Body: Sensory System (Eyes)
- Metal to Balance: Silver (supports eye health and improves vision)
- Ring Finger Placement: Index Finger – enhances eye health and improves night vision.

9. Nodule (Thyroid)

- System of the Body: Endocrine System (Thyroid)
- Metal to Balance: Copper (supports thyroid health and reduces inflammation)
- Ring Finger Placement: Middle Finger – supports endocrine health and thyroid function.

10. Nosebleeds (Epistaxis)

- System of the Body: Circulatory System
- Metal to Balance: Silver (calms and supports blood vessel health)
- Ring Finger Placement: Little Finger – supports nasal passage health and reduces bleeding.

Top Ten Common Conditions starting with "O"

1. Obesity

- System of the Body: Endocrine System (Metabolism)
- Metal to Balance: Copper (supports metabolic processes and weight management)
- Ring Finger Placement: Middle Finger – enhances metabolic health and supports weight regulation.

2. Obsessive-Compulsive Disorder (OCD)

- System of the Body: Nervous System
- Metal to Balance: Platinum (supports mental clarity and emotional balance)
- Ring Finger Placement: Thumb – influences brain function and mental health.

3. Osteoarthritis

- System of the Body: Musculoskeletal System (Joints)
- Metal to Balance: Copper (reduces inflammation and supports joint health)
- Ring Finger Placement: Index Finger – supports joint health and reduces pain.

4. Osteoporosis

- System of the Body: Skeletal System (Bones)
- Metal to Balance: Titanium (supports bone density and strength)
- Ring Finger Placement: Middle Finger – enhances bone health and structural integrity.

5. Otitis Media (Middle Ear Infection)

- System of the Body: Sensory System (Ears)
- Metal to Balance: Silver (antimicrobial and supports ear health)
- Ring Finger Placement: Index Finger – supports auditory function and reduces infection.

6. Otitis Externa (Swimmer's Ear)

- System of the Body: Sensory System (Ears)
- Metal to Balance: Silver (antimicrobial and supports ear health)
- Ring Finger Placement: Index Finger – supports ear health and reduces infection.

7. Osteomyelitis

- System of the Body: Skeletal System (Bones)
- Metal to Balance: Titanium (supports bone health and reduces infection)
- Ring Finger Placement: Middle Finger – enhances bone health and supports healing.

8. Oral Thrush

- System of the Body: Oral Health (Mouth)
- Metal to Balance: Silver (antimicrobial and supports oral health)
- Ring Finger Placement: Index Finger – supports oral health and reduces fungal infection.

9. Ovarian Cysts

- System of the Body: Reproductive System
- Metal to Balance: Gold (supports reproductive health and reduces cysts)
- Ring Finger Placement: Ring Finger – enhances reproductive health and reduces discomfort.

10. Osteomalacia

- System of the Body: Skeletal System (Bones)
- Metal to Balance: Titanium (supports bone strength and mineralization)
- Ring Finger Placement: Middle Finger – enhances bone health and supports structural integrity.

Top Ten Common Conditions starting with "P"

1. Parkinson's Disease

- System of the Body: Nervous System
- Metal to Balance: Platinum (supports neurological function and reduces symptoms)
- Ring Finger Placement: Thumb – enhances brain function and supports nerve health.

2. Pneumonia

- System of the Body: Respiratory System
- Metal to Balance: Silver (antimicrobial and supports respiratory health)
- Ring Finger Placement: Little Finger – supports lung health and reduces infection.

3. Psoriasis

- System of the Body: Integumentary System (Skin)
- Metal to Balance: Silver (reduces inflammation and supports skin health)
- Ring Finger Placement: Ring Finger – supports skin health and reduces symptoms.

4. Pancreatitis

- System of the Body: Digestive System (Pancreas)
- Metal to Balance: Copper (supports pancreatic health and reduces inflammation)
- Ring Finger Placement: Middle Finger – enhances digestive function and supports pancreatic health.

5. Peptic Ulcer

- System of the Body: Digestive System (Stomach)
- Metal to Balance: Copper (supports digestive health and reduces acidity)
- Ring Finger Placement: Middle Finger – supports stomach health and reduces ulcer symptoms.

6. Peripheral Neuropathy

- System of the Body: Nervous System
- Metal to Balance: Platinum (supports nerve health and reduces symptoms)
- Ring Finger Placement: Thumb – enhances nerve function and supports peripheral nerve health.

7. Phlebitis

- System of the Body: Circulatory System (Veins)
- Metal to Balance: Copper (reduces inflammation and supports vein health)
- Ring Finger Placement: Little Finger – supports venous health and reduces inflammation.

8. Polycystic Ovary Syndrome (PCOS)

- System of the Body: Reproductive System
- Metal to Balance: Gold (supports hormonal balance and reduces cysts)
- Ring Finger Placement: Ring Finger – enhances reproductive health and reduces symptoms.

9. Prostatitis

- System of the Body: Reproductive System (Prostate)
- Metal to Balance: Gold (supports prostate health and reduces inflammation)
- Ring Finger Placement: Ring Finger – supports prostate health and reduces discomfort.

10. Psoriatic Arthritis

- System of the Body: Musculoskeletal System (Joints)
- Metal to Balance: Copper (reduces inflammation and supports joint health)
- Ring Finger Placement: Index Finger – supports joint health and reduces pain.

Top Ten Common Conditions starting with "Q"

1. Quinsy (Peritonsillar Abscess)

- System of the Body: Respiratory System (Throat)
- Metal to Balance: Silver (antimicrobial and supports respiratory health)
- Ring Finger Placement: Little Finger – supports throat health and reduces infection.

2. Quadriplegia

- System of the Body: Nervous System
- Metal to Balance: Platinum (supports neurological function and recovery)
- Ring Finger Placement: Thumb – enhances nerve function and supports spinal health.

3. Q Fever

- System of the Body: Immune System
- Metal to Balance: Silver (antimicrobial and supports immune function)
- Ring Finger Placement: Index Finger – supports immune response and reduces bacterial infection.

4. Quickening (Fetal Movement)

- System of the Body: Reproductive System
- Metal to Balance: Gold (supports reproductive health and vitality)
- Ring Finger Placement: Ring Finger – enhances maternal health and supports fetal development.

5. Quivering (Tremors)

- System of the Body: Nervous System
- Metal to Balance: Platinum (supports neurological function and reduces tremors)
- Ring Finger Placement: Thumb – enhances brain function and supports motor control.

6. Quadriceps Strain

- System of the Body: Musculoskeletal System (Muscles)
- Metal to Balance: Copper (supports muscle health and reduces inflammation)
- Ring Finger Placement: Index Finger – supports muscle recovery and reduces pain.

7. Quarantine (Infectious Disease Management)

- System of the Body: Immune System
- Metal to Balance: Silver (supports immune function and reduces infection spread)
- Ring Finger Placement: Index Finger – enhances immune response and supports infection control.

8. Quaternary Ammonium Compounds Poisoning

- System of the Body: Digestive System
- Metal to Balance: Copper (supports detoxification and digestive health)
- Ring Finger Placement: Middle Finger – supports liver function and detoxification.

9. Quinidine Toxicity

- System of the Body: Circulatory System (Heart)
- Metal to Balance: Gold (supports heart health and reduces toxicity effects)
- Ring Finger Placement: Ring Finger – enhances cardiovascular health and supports heart function.

10. Quick Pulse (Tachycardia)

- System of the Body: Circulatory System
- Metal to Balance: Silver (calms and supports heart health)
- Ring Finger Placement: Middle Finger – enhances heart health and supports circulation

Top Ten Common Conditions starting with "R"

1. Rheumatoid Arthritis

- System of the Body: Musculoskeletal System (Joints)
- Metal to Balance: Copper (reduces inflammation and supports joint health)
- Ring Finger Placement: Index Finger – supports joint health and reduces pain.

2. Rosacea

- System of the Body: Integumentary System (Skin)
- Metal to Balance: Silver (reduces inflammation and supports skin health)
- Ring Finger Placement: Ring Finger – supports skin health and reduces symptoms.

3. Rhinitis (Hay Fever)

- System of the Body: Respiratory System
- Metal to Balance: Stainless Steel (supports immune function and reduces inflammation)
- Ring Finger Placement: Index Finger – enhances immune response and reduces allergy symptoms.

4. Restless Leg Syndrome

- System of the Body: Nervous System
- Metal to Balance: Platinum (supports neurological function and reduces symptoms)
- Ring Finger Placement: Thumb – enhances nerve function and supports motor control.

5. Rheumatic Fever

- System of the Body: Circulatory System
- Metal to Balance: Gold (supports heart health and reduces inflammation)
- Ring Finger Placement: Ring Finger – enhances cardiovascular health and supports heart function.

6. Retinal Detachment

- System of the Body: Sensory System (Eyes)
- Metal to Balance: Silver (supports eye health and reduces inflammation)
- Ring Finger Placement: Index Finger – supports retinal health and vision.

7. Rickets

- System of the Body: Skeletal System (Bones)
- Metal to Balance: Titanium (supports bone health and mineralization)
- Ring Finger Placement: Middle Finger – enhances bone health and supports structural integrity.

8. Ringworm (Tinea)

- System of the Body: Integumentary System (Skin)
- Metal to Balance: Silver (antimicrobial and supports skin health)
- Ring Finger Placement: Ring Finger – supports skin health and reduces fungal infection.

9. Rotator Cuff Injury

- System of the Body: Musculoskeletal System (Shoulder)
- Metal to Balance: Copper (reduces inflammation and supports muscle and joint health)
- Ring Finger Placement: Index Finger – supports shoulder health and reduces pain.

10. Raynaud's Disease

- System of the Body: Circulatory System
- Metal to Balance: Gold (supports circulation and reduces symptoms)
- Ring Finger Placement: Ring Finger – enhances blood flow and supports vascular health.

Top Ten Common Conditions starting with "S"

1. Sciatica

- System of the Body: Nervous System
- Metal to Balance: Platinum (supports nerve health and reduces pain)
- Ring Finger Placement: Thumb – enhances nerve function and reduces sciatic pain.

2. Scoliosis

- System of the Body: Musculoskeletal System (Spine)
- Metal to Balance: Titanium (supports spinal health and alignment)
- Ring Finger Placement: Middle Finger – enhances spinal health and supports structural integrity.

3. Sinusitis

- System of the Body: Respiratory System (Sinuses)
- Metal to Balance: Silver (reduces inflammation and supports respiratory health)
- Ring Finger Placement: Little Finger – supports sinus health and reduces infection.

4. Skin Cancer

- System of the Body: Integumentary System (Skin)
- Metal to Balance: Silver (supports skin health and reduces inflammation)
- Ring Finger Placement: Ring Finger – supports skin health and reduces cancerous growths.

5. Sleep Apnea

- System of the Body: Respiratory System
- Metal to Balance: Silver (supports respiratory function and reduces inflammation)
- Ring Finger Placement: Little Finger – enhances respiratory health and supports better sleep.

6. Sore Throat (Pharyngitis)

- System of the Body: Respiratory System (Throat)
- Metal to Balance: Silver (antimicrobial and supports throat health)
- Ring Finger Placement: Little Finger – supports throat health and reduces inflammation.

7. Sprains

- System of the Body: Musculoskeletal System (Joints)
- Metal to Balance: Copper (reduces inflammation and supports joint health)
- Ring Finger Placement: Index Finger – supports joint health and reduces pain.

8. Stomach Ulcers

- System of the Body: Digestive System (Stomach)
- Metal to Balance: Copper (supports digestive health and reduces acidity)
- Ring Finger Placement: Middle Finger – supports stomach health and reduces ulcer symptoms.

9. Stroke

- System of the Body: Circulatory System
- Metal to Balance: Platinum (supports brain health and recovery)
- Ring Finger Placement: Thumb – enhances brain function and supports recovery post-stroke.

10. Systemic Lupus Erythematosus (SLE)

- System of the Body: Immune System
- Metal to Balance: Silver (reduces inflammation and supports immune function)
- Ring Finger Placement: Index Finger – enhances immune response and reduces autoimmune symptoms.

Top Ten Common Conditions starting with "T"

1. Tendonitis

- System of the Body: Musculoskeletal System (Tendons)
- Metal to Balance: Copper (reduces inflammation and supports tendon health)
- Ring Finger Placement: Index Finger – supports tendon health and reduces pain.

2. Tetanus

- System of the Body: Nervous System
- Metal to Balance: Platinum (supports nerve health and reduces muscle spasms)
- Ring Finger Placement: Thumb – enhances nerve function and reduces symptoms.

3. Thyroiditis

- System of the Body: Endocrine System (Thyroid)
- Metal to Balance: Copper (supports thyroid health and reduces inflammation)
- Ring Finger Placement: Middle Finger – enhances endocrine function and supports thyroid health.

4. Tinnitus

- System of the Body: Sensory System (Ears)
- Metal to Balance: Silver (supports auditory health and reduces inflammation)
- Ring Finger Placement: Index Finger – enhances ear health and reduces ringing.

5. Tonsillitis

- System of the Body: Respiratory System (Throat)
- Metal to Balance: Silver (antimicrobial and supports throat health)
- Ring Finger Placement: Little Finger – supports throat health and reduces inflammation.

6. Tuberculosis (TB)

- System of the Body: Respiratory System
- Metal to Balance: Silver (antimicrobial and supports respiratory health)
- Ring Finger Placement: Little Finger – enhances lung health and reduces infection.

7. Tachycardia

- System of the Body: Circulatory System
- Metal to Balance: Gold (energizes and supports heart health)
- Ring Finger Placement: Ring Finger – enhances heart function and reduces heart rate.

8. Thrombophlebitis

- System of the Body: Circulatory System (Veins)
- Metal to Balance: Copper (reduces inflammation and supports vein health)
- Ring Finger Placement: Little Finger – supports venous health and reduces inflammation.

9. Toxoplasmosis

- System of the Body: Immune System
- Metal to Balance: Silver (supports immune function and reduces infection)
- Ring Finger Placement: Index Finger – enhances immune response and reduces parasitic infection.

10. Trichomoniasis

- System of the Body: Reproductive System
- Metal to Balance: Gold (supports reproductive health and reduces infection)
- Ring Finger Placement: Ring Finger – enhances reproductive health and reduces symptoms.

Top Ten Common Conditions starting with "U"

1. Ulcerative Colitis

- System of the Body: Digestive System (Colon)
- Metal to Balance: Copper (supports digestive health and reduces inflammation)
- Ring Finger Placement: Middle Finger – supports intestinal health and reduces symptoms.

2. Urinary Tract Infection (UTI)

- System of the Body: Urinary System
- Metal to Balance: Cobalt (supports urinary health and reduces infection)
- Ring Finger Placement: Index Finger – supports bladder health and reduces symptoms.

3. Urticaria (Hives)

- System of the Body: Integumentary System (Skin)
- Metal to Balance: Silver (reduces inflammation and supports skin health)
- Ring Finger Placement: Ring Finger – supports skin health and reduces itching.

4. Uterine Fibroids

- System of the Body: Reproductive System
- Metal to Balance: Gold (supports reproductive health and reduces growths)
- Ring Finger Placement: Ring Finger – enhances reproductive health and reduces discomfort.

5. Ulcers (Peptic Ulcers)

- System of the Body: Digestive System (Stomach)
- Metal to Balance: Copper (supports digestive health and reduces acidity)
- Ring Finger Placement: Middle Finger – supports stomach health and reduces ulcer symptoms.

6. Upper Respiratory Tract Infection

- System of the Body: Respiratory System
- Metal to Balance: Silver (supports respiratory health and reduces infection)
- Ring Finger Placement: Little Finger – enhances respiratory health and reduces symptoms.

7. Uveitis

- System of the Body: Sensory System (Eyes)
- Metal to Balance: Silver (reduces inflammation and supports eye health)
- Ring Finger Placement: Index Finger – supports eye health and reduces inflammation.

8. Urolithiasis (Kidney Stones)

- System of the Body: Urinary System (Kidneys)
- Metal to Balance: Cobalt (supports kidney health and reduces stone formation)
- Ring Finger Placement: Index Finger – supports kidney function and urinary health.

9. Umbilical Hernia

- System of the Body: Musculoskeletal System (Abdomen)
- Metal to Balance: Titanium (supports muscle health and reduces discomfort)
- Ring Finger Placement: Middle Finger – supports abdominal health and reduces hernia symptoms.

10. Unstable Angina

- System of the Body: Circulatory System (Heart)
- Metal to Balance: Gold (supports heart health and reduces pain)
- Ring Finger Placement: Ring Finger – enhances cardiovascular health and reduces symptoms.

Top Ten Common Conditions starting with "V"

1. Varicose Veins

- System of the Body: Circulatory System
- Metal to Balance: Copper (improves circulation and reduces inflammation)
- Ring Finger Placement: Little Finger – supports venous circulation and reduces swelling.

2. Vaginitis

- System of the Body: Reproductive System
- Metal to Balance: Gold (supports reproductive health and reduces infection)
- Ring Finger Placement: Ring Finger – enhances reproductive health and reduces symptoms.

3. Vertigo

- System of the Body: Nervous System
- Metal to Balance: Platinum (supports neurological function and reduces dizziness)
- Ring Finger Placement: Thumb – enhances brain function and supports balance.

4. Viral Infections

- System of the Body: Immune System
- Metal to Balance: Silver (antimicrobial and supports immune function)
- Ring Finger Placement: Index Finger – enhances immune response and reduces viral activity.

5. Vitiligo

- System of the Body: Integumentary System (Skin)
- Metal to Balance: Silver (supports skin health and reduces inflammation)
- Ring Finger Placement: Ring Finger – supports skin health and reduces symptoms.

6. Vulvodynia

- System of the Body: Reproductive System
- Metal to Balance: Gold (supports reproductive health and reduces pain)
- Ring Finger Placement: Ring Finger – enhances reproductive health and reduces discomfort.

7. Varicocele

- System of the Body: Reproductive System
- Metal to Balance: Gold (supports reproductive health and reduces swelling)
- Ring Finger Placement: Ring Finger – enhances reproductive health and reduces symptoms.

8. Vasculitis

- System of the Body: Circulatory System
- Metal to Balance: Copper (reduces inflammation and supports vascular health)
- Ring Finger Placement: Little Finger – supports blood vessel health and reduces inflammation.

9. Venous Thromboembolism (VTE)

- System of the Body: Circulatory System
- Metal to Balance: Copper (improves circulation and reduces clotting)
- Ring Finger Placement: Little Finger – supports venous circulation and reduces risk of clots.

10. Vulvovaginal Candidiasis

- System of the Body: Reproductive System
- Metal to Balance: Gold (supports reproductive health and reduces infection)
- Ring Finger Placement: Ring Finger – enhances reproductive health and reduces symptoms.

Top Ten Common Conditions starting with "W"

1. Warts

- System of the Body: Integumentary System (Skin)
- Metal to Balance: Silver (antimicrobial and supports skin health)
- Ring Finger Placement: Ring Finger – supports skin health and reduces wart growth.

2. Whooping Cough (Pertussis)

- System of the Body: Respiratory System
- Metal to Balance: Silver (supports respiratory health and reduces infection)
- Ring Finger Placement: Little Finger – supports lung health and reduces symptoms.

3. Whiplash

- System of the Body: Musculoskeletal System (Neck)
- Metal to Balance: Copper (reduces inflammation and supports muscle health)
- Ring Finger Placement: Index Finger – supports neck health and reduces pain.

4. Wilson's Disease

- System of the Body: Hepatic System (Liver)
- Metal to Balance: Copper (supports liver health and reduces copper accumulation)
- Ring Finger Placement: Middle Finger – enhances liver function and supports detoxification.

5. Wound Healing

- System of the Body: Integumentary System (Skin)
- Metal to Balance: Silver (supports skin healing and reduces infection)
- Ring Finger Placement: Ring Finger – supports skin health and promotes faster healing.

6. Wegener's Granulomatosis (Granulomatosis with Polyangiitis)

- System of the Body: Immune System
- Metal to Balance: Silver (reduces inflammation and supports immune function)
- Ring Finger Placement: Index Finger – enhances immune response and reduces autoimmune symptoms.

7. Wrist Pain

- System of the Body: Musculoskeletal System (Wrist)
- Metal to Balance: Copper (reduces inflammation and supports joint health)
- Ring Finger Placement: Index Finger – supports wrist health and reduces pain.

8. Wolff-Parkinson-White Syndrome

- System of the Body: Circulatory System (Heart)
- Metal to Balance: Gold (supports heart health and reduces symptoms)
- Ring Finger Placement: Ring Finger – enhances cardiovascular health and supports heart function.

9. Wheezing

- System of the Body: Respiratory System
- Metal to Balance: Silver (supports respiratory health and reduces inflammation)
- Ring Finger Placement: Little Finger – supports lung health and reduces symptoms.

10. Weakness

- System of the Body: Nervous System
- Metal to Balance: Platinum (supports neurological function and reduces fatigue)
- Ring Finger Placement: Thumb – enhances nerve function and supports overall vitality.

Top Ten Common Conditions starting with "X"

1. Xerophthalmia

- System of the Body: Sensory System (Eyes)
- Metal to Balance: Silver (supports eye health and reduces dryness)
- Ring Finger Placement: Index Finger – enhances eye health and reduces symptoms.

2. Xeroderma

- System of the Body: Integumentary System (Skin)
- Metal to Balance: Silver (supports skin health and reduces dryness)
- Ring Finger Placement: Ring Finger – supports skin health and reduces symptoms.

3. Xanthoma

- System of the Body: Integumentary System (Skin)
- Metal to Balance: Silver (supports skin health and reduces lipid deposits)
- Ring Finger Placement: Ring Finger – supports skin health and reduces symptoms.

4. X-linked Agammaglobulinemia

- System of the Body: Immune System
- Metal to Balance: Silver (supports immune function and reduces infection)
- Ring Finger Placement: Index Finger – enhances immune response and reduces symptoms.

5. Xerosis

- System of the Body: Integumentary System (Skin)
- Metal to Balance: Silver (supports skin health and reduces dryness)
- Ring Finger Placement: Ring Finger – supports skin health and reduces symptoms.

6. Xanthelasma

- System of the Body: Integumentary System (Skin)
- Metal to Balance: Silver (supports skin health and reduces cholesterol deposits)
- Ring Finger Placement: Ring Finger – supports skin health and reduces symptoms.

7. Xenophobia

- System of the Body: Nervous System
- Metal to Balance: Platinum (supports mental clarity and reduces anxiety)
- Ring Finger Placement: Thumb – enhances brain function and reduces anxiety.

8. X-linked Ichthyosis

- System of the Body: Integumentary System (Skin)
- Metal to Balance: Silver (supports skin health and reduces scaling)
- Ring Finger Placement: Ring Finger – supports skin health and reduces symptoms.

9. Xanthinuria

- System of the Body: Urinary System
- Metal to Balance: Copper (supports kidney function and reduces xanthine accumulation)
- Ring Finger Placement: Index Finger – supports kidney health and reduces symptoms.

10. Xerostomia (Dry Mouth)

- System of the Body: Oral Health
- Metal to Balance: Silver (supports salivary gland function and reduces dryness)
- Ring Finger Placement: Index Finger – supports oral health and reduces symptoms.

Top Ten Common Conditions starting with "Y"

1. Yeast Infection (Candidiasis)

- System of the Body: Reproductive System
- Metal to Balance: Gold (supports reproductive health and reduces infection)
- Ring Finger Placement: Ring Finger – enhances reproductive health and reduces symptoms.

2. Yellow Fever

- System of the Body: Immune System
- Metal to Balance: Silver (supports immune function and reduces viral activity)
- Ring Finger Placement: Index Finger – enhances immune response and reduces symptoms.

3. Yersiniosis

- System of the Body: Digestive System
- Metal to Balance: Silver (supports digestive health and reduces bacterial infection)
- Ring Finger Placement: Middle Finger – enhances digestive health and reduces symptoms.

4. Young-Onset Parkinson's Disease

- System of the Body: Nervous System
- Metal to Balance: Platinum (supports neurological function and reduces symptoms)
- Ring Finger Placement: Thumb – enhances brain function and supports nerve health.

5. Yttrium Exposure (Toxicity)

- System of the Body: Various (depends on exposure)
- Metal to Balance: Copper (supports detoxification and reduces toxicity)
- Ring Finger Placement: Middle Finger – supports liver and kidney function for detoxification.

6. Yolk Sac Tumor

- System of the Body: Reproductive System
- Metal to Balance: Gold (supports reproductive health and reduces tumor growth)
- Ring Finger Placement: Ring Finger – enhances reproductive health and reduces symptoms.

7. Yersinia Enterocolitica Infection

- System of the Body: Digestive System
- Metal to Balance: Silver (supports immune function and reduces bacterial infection)
- Ring Finger Placement: Middle Finger – supports digestive health and reduces symptoms.

8. Yellow Nail Syndrome

- System of the Body: Integumentary System (Nails)
- Metal to Balance: Silver (supports nail health and reduces discoloration)
- Ring Finger Placement: Ring Finger – enhances nail health and reduces symptoms.

9. Yusho Disease

- System of the Body: Various (due to PCB exposure)
- Metal to Balance: Copper (supports detoxification and reduces symptoms)
- Ring Finger Placement: Middle Finger – supports liver and kidney function for detoxification.

10. Yamaguchi Syndrome

- System of the Body: Cardiovascular System
- Metal to Balance: Gold (supports heart health and reduces symptoms)
- Ring Finger Placement: Ring Finger – enhances cardiovascular health and reduces symptoms.

Top Ten Common Conditions starting with "Z"

1. Zinc Deficiency

- System of the Body: Various (Immune, Skin, Digestive)
- Metal to Balance: Zinc (supports immune function, skin health, and metabolism)
- Metal to Balance: Silver (supports immune function, skin health, and metabolism)
- Ring Finger Placement: Middle Finger – enhances overall health and reduces deficiency symptoms.

2. Zollinger-Ellison Syndrome

- System of the Body: Digestive System (Stomach)
- Metal to Balance: Copper (supports digestive health and reduces acid production)
- Ring Finger Placement: Middle Finger – supports stomach health and reduces ulcer symptoms.

3. Zika Virus

- System of the Body: Immune System
- Metal to Balance: Silver (supports immune function and reduces viral activity)
- Ring Finger Placement: Index Finger – enhances immune response and reduces symptoms.

4. Zinc Toxicity

- System of the Body: Various (depends on exposure)
- Metal to Balance: Copper (supports detoxification and reduces toxicity)
- Ring Finger Placement: Middle Finger – supports liver and kidney function for detoxification.

5. Zoster (Shingles)

- System of the Body: Immune System
- Metal to Balance: Silver (supports immune function and reduces viral activity)
- Ring Finger Placement: Index Finger – enhances immune response and reduces symptoms.

6. Zoonotic Diseases

- System of the Body: Immune System
- Metal to Balance: Silver (supports immune function and reduces infection)
- Ring Finger Placement: Index Finger – supports immune response and reduces transmission.

7. Zenker's Diverticulum

- System of the Body: Digestive System (Esophagus)
- Metal to Balance: Copper (supports esophageal health and reduces symptoms)
- Ring Finger Placement: Middle Finger – supports digestive health and reduces symptoms.

8. Zygomycosis (Mucormycosis)

- System of the Body: Immune System
- Metal to Balance: Silver (antifungal and supports immune function)
- Ring Finger Placement: Index Finger – enhances immune response and reduces fungal infection.

9. Zinc Overload

- System of the Body: Various (depends on exposure)
- Metal to Balance: Copper (supports detoxification and reduces symptoms)
- Ring Finger Placement: Middle Finger – supports liver and kidney function for detoxification.

10. Zygomatic Fracture

- System of the Body: Musculoskeletal System (Face)
- Metal to Balance: Titanium (supports bone healing and strength)
- Ring Finger Placement: Middle Finger – supports facial bone health and recovery.

Appendices

Case Studies

Case Study: Weight Loss

Background

Sarah, a 35-year-old woman, has struggled with weight loss for several years. Despite trying various diets and exercise programs, she has found it difficult to lose weight and keep it off. She decides to explore holistic approaches and learns about the potential benefits of metal ring balancing from Dr. Constance Santego's book.

Initial Assessment

Sarah visits Dr. Constance for a personalized session. During the session, Dr. Constance performs a muscle test to determine the optimal metal and finger placement for supporting Sarah's weight loss journey.

Muscle Testing Procedure

1. Preparation: Sarah ensures she is well-hydrated and in a calm, relaxed state.
2. Establishing a Baseline: Dr. Constance uses the Arm method to establish Sarah's baseline strength.

3. Testing for Metals: Dr. Constance tests the metals, including gold, silver, copper, and nickel, to determine which one provides the strongest response for weight loss.
4. Testing Finger Placement: Once nickel shows the strongest response, Dr. Constance tests various fingers to identify the optimal placement.

Results

Metal: Nickel

Finger Placement: Middle Finger (Third Finger)

Plan and Implementation

Dr. Constance explains that nickel's properties of strength and durability can support Sarah's muscular health and overall physical endurance, which are crucial for an effective weight loss program. Wearing a nickel ring on the middle finger is believed to promote balance, strength, and stability, aligning with Sarah's weight loss goals.

Weekly Monitoring and Adjustments

Sarah wears the nickel ring on her middle finger daily and follows up with Dr. Constance weekly. During these sessions, they re-evaluate the effectiveness of the ring and make any necessary adjustments to the duration and placement.

Results After Three Months

- Weight Loss: Sarah loses 15 pounds.
- Improved Endurance: Sarah reports increased stamina during her workouts.
- Enhanced Muscle Strength: She experiences better muscle tone and strength.

- Emotional Stability: Sarah feels more balanced and motivated, which helps her stick to her weight loss plan.

Conclusion

Sarah's case demonstrates the potential benefits of using metal ring balancing to support weight loss. By combining traditional holistic practices with modern techniques, Sarah was able to enhance her physical and emotional well-being, leading to successful weight loss and improved overall health. This case study highlights the effectiveness of personalized metal ring therapy in achieving health and wellness goals.

Case Study: Financial Success

Background

John, a 42-year-old businessman, has been experiencing financial difficulties for the past few years. Despite working hard and having a solid business plan, he finds it challenging to achieve financial stability and success. He decides to explore holistic approaches and learns about the potential benefits of metal ring balancing from Dr. Constance Santego's book.

Initial Assessment

John schedules a session with Dr. Constance for a personalized muscle testing session to determine the optimal metal and finger placement to support his financial success.

Muscle Testing Procedure

1. Preparation: John ensures he is well-hydrated and in a calm, relaxed state.

2. Establishing a Baseline: Dr. Constance uses the O-Ring method to establish John's baseline strength.
3. Testing for Metals: Dr. Constance tests several metals, including gold, silver, copper, and platinum, to determine which one provides the strongest response for financial success.
4. Testing Finger Placement: Once gold shows the strongest response, Dr. Constance tests various fingers to identify the optimal placement.

Results

Metal: Gold

Finger Placement: Ring Finger (Fourth Finger)

Plan and Implementation

Dr. Constance explains that gold's properties of attracting and concentrating energy can support John's goals for financial success. Wearing a gold ring on the ring finger, which is associated with stability and balance, is believed to enhance John's confidence, decision-making, and overall financial prosperity.

Weekly Monitoring and Adjustments

John wears the gold ring on his ring finger daily and follows up with Dr. Constance weekly. During these sessions, they re-evaluate the effectiveness of the ring and make any necessary adjustments to the duration and placement.

Results After Three Months

- Increased Financial Opportunities: John reports several new business opportunities and partnerships.
- Improved Decision-Making: John feels more confident and decisive in his business dealings.

- Enhanced Prosperity: John experiences an overall improvement in his financial situation, including increased revenue and savings.
- Emotional Stability: John feels more balanced and less stressed about financial matters, which contributes to better focus and productivity.

Conclusion

John's case demonstrates the potential benefits of using metal ring balancing to support financial success. By combining traditional holistic practices with modern techniques, John was able to enhance his confidence, attract new opportunities, and achieve greater financial stability. This case study highlights the effectiveness of personalized metal ring therapy in achieving financial goals and overall well-being.

Case Study: Relationship Success via Zoom

Background

Emily, a 30-year-old professional, has been struggling with her relationships, both romantic and platonic. Despite her best efforts, she finds it difficult to maintain meaningful and harmonious connections. She decides to explore holistic approaches and learns about the potential benefits of metal ring balancing from Dr. Constance Santego's book. Due to geographical constraints, Emily opts for a Zoom session with Dr. Constance.

Initial Assessment

Emily schedules a Zoom session with Dr. Constance for a personalized muscle testing session to determine the optimal metal and finger placement to support her relationship success.

Muscle Testing Procedure

1. Preparation: Emily ensures she is well-hydrated and in a calm, relaxed state.
2. Establishing a Baseline: Dr. Constance instructs Emily to perform the Body method on herself to establish her baseline strength.
3. Testing for Metals: Dr. Constance guides Emily through testing several metals, including gold, silver, copper, and platinum, to determine which one provides the strongest response for relationship success.
4. Testing Finger Placement: Once gold shows the strongest response, Dr. Constance instructs Emily to test various fingers to identify the optimal placement.

Results

Metal: Gold

Finger Placement: Little Finger (Fifth Finger)

Plan and Implementation

Dr. Constance explains that gold's properties of attracting positive energy and fostering emotional stability can support Emily's goals for relationship success. Wearing a gold ring on the little finger, which is associated with emotional clarity and communication, is believed to enhance Emily's ability to connect with others and maintain harmonious relationships.

Weekly Monitoring and Adjustments

Emily wears the gold ring on her little finger daily and follows up with Dr. Constance via Zoom on a weekly basis. During these sessions, they re-evaluate the effectiveness of the ring and make any necessary adjustments to the duration and placement.

Results After Three Months

- Improved Communication: Emily reports better communication and understanding in her relationships.
- Strengthened Connections: Emily experiences deeper and more meaningful connections with both friends and romantic partners.
- Enhanced Emotional Stability: Emily feels more emotionally balanced and less reactive, contributing to healthier interactions.
- Increased Harmony: Overall, Emily finds her relationships to be more harmonious and fulfilling.

Conclusion

Emily's case demonstrates the potential benefits of using metal ring balancing to support relationship success. By combining traditional holistic practices with modern techniques via Zoom, Emily was able to enhance her communication skills, emotional stability, and overall relationship health. This case study highlights the effectiveness of personalized metal ring therapy in achieving harmonious and meaningful relationships.

Case Study: Supportive Therapy for Cancer

Background

David, a 55-year-old man, was diagnosed with cancer and has been undergoing conventional treatments such as chemotherapy and radiation. Seeking additional support for his overall well-being and recovery, David learns about the potential benefits of metal ring balancing from Dr. Constance Santego's book. He decides to explore this holistic approach to complement his ongoing medical treatments.

Initial Assessment

David schedules a session with Dr. Constance for a personalized muscle testing session to determine the optimal metal and finger placement to support his cancer treatment and overall health.

Muscle Testing Procedure

1. Preparation: David ensures he is well-hydrated and in a calm, relaxed state.
2. Establishing a Baseline: Dr. Constance uses the O-Ring method to establish David's baseline strength.
3. Testing for Metals: Dr. Constance tests several metals, including gold, silver, platinum, and titanium, to determine which one provides the strongest supportive response for David's condition.
4. Testing Finger Placement: Once platinum shows the strongest response, Dr. Constance tests various fingers to identify the optimal placement.

Results

Metal: Platinum

Finger Placement: Index Finger (Second Finger)

Plan and Implementation

Dr. Constance explains that platinum's properties of enhancing cell repair and supporting the immune system can be beneficial for David's overall health during cancer treatment. Wearing a platinum ring on the index finger, which is associated with strength and self-empowerment, is believed to enhance David's resilience and support his body's healing processes.

Weekly Monitoring and Adjustments

David wears the platinum ring on his index finger daily and follows up with Dr. Constance weekly. During these sessions, they re-evaluate the effectiveness of the ring and make any necessary adjustments to the duration and placement.

Results After Three Months

- Improved Energy Levels: David reports higher energy levels and less fatigue, allowing him to better cope with his treatments.
- Enhanced Immune Function: David experiences fewer infections and quicker recovery times between chemotherapy sessions.
- Better Mood and Outlook: David feels more positive and emotionally balanced, which helps him stay motivated and resilient throughout his treatment.
- Supportive Healing: Overall, David finds that the platinum ring provides a supportive boost to his conventional cancer treatments, contributing to his sense of well-being and recovery.

Conclusion

David's case demonstrates the potential benefits of using metal ring balancing as a complementary therapy for cancer treatment. By combining traditional holistic practices with modern techniques, David was able to enhance his energy levels, immune function, and overall emotional well-being. This case study highlights the effectiveness of personalized metal ring therapy in providing supportive care during challenging medical treatments.

Case Study: Recovery & Prevention of Heart Attack

Background

Mark, a 60-year-old man, recently experienced a heart attack and has been undergoing conventional medical treatments to aid his recovery. Seeking additional support for his heart health and prevention of future incidents, Mark learns about the potential benefits of metal ring balancing from Dr. Constance Santego's book. He decides to explore this holistic approach to complement his ongoing medical care.

Initial Assessment

Mark schedules a session with Dr. Constance for a personalized muscle testing session to determine the optimal metal and finger placement to support his heart health and recovery.

Muscle Testing Procedure

1. Preparation: Mark ensures he is well-hydrated and in a calm, relaxed state.
2. Establishing a Baseline: Dr. Constance uses the O-Ring method to establish Mark's baseline strength.
3. Testing for Metals: Dr. Constance tests several metals, including gold, silver, and copper, to determine which one provides the strongest supportive response for Mark's heart health.
4. Testing Finger Placement: Once gold shows the strongest response, Dr. Constance tests various fingers to identify the optimal placement.

Results

> Metal: Gold
>
> Finger Placement: Ring Finger (Fourth Finger)

Plan and Implementation

Dr. Constance explains that gold's properties of enhancing blood circulation and emotional stability can be beneficial for Mark's heart health. Wearing a gold ring on the ring finger, which is associated with the heart meridian and emotional stability, is believed to support heart function and promote a sense of calm and balance.

Weekly Monitoring and Adjustments

Mark wears the gold ring on his ring finger daily and follows up with Dr. Constance weekly. During these sessions, they re-evaluate the effectiveness of the ring and make any necessary adjustments to the duration and placement.

Results After Three Months

- Improved Circulation: Mark reports better blood circulation and fewer episodes of chest discomfort.
- Enhanced Emotional Stability: Mark feels more emotionally balanced and less anxious, which helps reduce stress on his heart.
- Increased Energy Levels: Mark experiences higher energy levels and improved stamina, allowing him to engage in light physical activities recommended by his doctor.
- Preventive Support: Overall, Mark finds that wearing the gold ring provides supportive care that complements his conventional treatments, helping to prevent future heart issues.

Conclusion

Mark's case demonstrates the potential benefits of using metal ring balancing as a complementary therapy for heart attack recovery and prevention. By combining traditional holistic practices with modern techniques, Mark was able to enhance his heart health, improve his emotional stability, and support his overall recovery. This case study highlights the effectiveness of personalized metal ring therapy in providing supportive care for heart health and preventing future incidents.

TRUE STORIES

"My husband had a thick gold chain that he used to wear, and one day, he decided to put it on our dog. To our surprise, the dog absolutely loved the gold chain and always wanted to wear it. Seeing how much he liked it, I bought a gold-colored chain for the dog. However, to my astonishment, he hated the fake gold chain and constantly tried to take it off. But whenever my husband put his real gold chain on the dog, he was perfectly happy and content. This experience proved to me that metals do make a difference, even to a dog who presumably doesn't know what he's wearing—or does he?"

DIANE

"I had a client call and told me that her son had been in two car accidents within a few days. I asked if anything significant had changed in his life just before the accidents. She mentioned that the only change was that he had gotten a tongue ring. I suggested he consider removing it or muscle test the ring and changing it to gold or silver."

CONNIE

Where to Purchase Metal Rings

Purchasing metal rings for health benefits or simply as jewelry can be done through various reputable retailers, both online and in physical stores. Here are some recommended sources for purchasing rings made of cobalt, palladium, titanium, and stainless steel:

ONLINE RETAILERS
Amazon:

- Amazon offers a wide range of metal rings, including those made from cobalt, palladium, titanium, and stainless steel. You can find various designs and price ranges, often with customer reviews to guide your purchase.
- https://www.amazon.ca/

Etsy:

- Etsy is a marketplace for handmade and vintage items. Many independent jewelers sell custom-made metal rings, including cobalt, palladium, titanium, and stainless steel rings.
- https://www.etsy.com/

Physical Stores, Specialty Stores, and Local Jewelers:

> Visiting local jewelry stores can provide personalized service and the opportunity to see and try on rings before purchasing. Many local jewelers can also custom-make rings using specific metals like cobalt, palladium, titanium, and stainless steel.

When purchasing metal rings for health benefits or as jewelry, it is important to choose reputable retailers that provide high-quality products. Whether you prefer shopping online or in physical stores, there are many options available for acquiring rings made from cobalt, palladium, titanium, and stainless steel. Always ensure that the seller offers detailed product information and reviews, and consider custom options if you have specific design preferences.

Ring Size and Meridian Stimulation

When selecting a metal ring for health purposes, it is beneficial to choose a size that is slightly larger than your usual ring size. This allows you to turn or spin the ring on your finger, which helps to stimulate the corresponding meridian points.

SIZE:

> Optimal Fit: Select a ring size that is slightly bigger than your regular fit. This enables the ring to move freely on your finger without being too loose.

> Meridian Stimulation: The ability to turn or spin the ring enhances stimulation of the meridian points located on the fingers. This movement can help activate and balance the energy flow in the associated meridians, promoting better health benefits.

> Comfort and Functionality: A slightly larger ring ensures comfort and allows for easy adjustment throughout the day, preventing any discomfort or restriction.

By choosing the right ring size and allowing for movement, you can maximize the therapeutic benefits of the metal ring and effectively support the health of your body's systems.

APPROXIMATE PRICES FOR METAL RINGS (SIZE 10) IN 2024

- Gold:
  - o 14k Gold Ring: Approximately $300 - $500
  - o 18k Gold Ring: Approximately $400 - $700
  - o 24k Gold Ring: Approximately $700 - $1,000
- Silver:
  - o Sterling Silver Ring: Approximately $20 - $50
- Copper:
  - o Copper Ring: Approximately $10 - $30
- Platinum:
  - o Platinum Ring: Approximately $800 - $1,200
- Titanium:
  - o Titanium Ring: Approximately $30 - $100
- Nickel:
  - o Nickel Ring: Approximately $10 - $25
- Stainless Steel:
  - o Stainless Steel Ring: Approximately $10 - $50
- Cobalt:
  - o Cobalt Ring: Approximately $50 - $150
- Palladium:
  - o Palladium Ring: Approximately $600 - $900

Reference Charts

Metals and Their Associated Properties

Metal	Properties	Benefits
Gold	Anti-inflammatory, hormonal balance, emotional stability	Reduces inflammation, supports hormonal balance, enhances emotional well-being
Silver	Antimicrobial, anti-inflammatory, skin health	Prevents infections, reduces skin inflammation, promotes wound healing
Copper	Anti-inflammatory, pain relief, immune support	Reduces joint pain, supports immune function, enhances skin health
Platinum	Mental clarity, emotional stability, anti-aging	Enhances cognitive function, reduces stress, promotes youthful skin
Titanium	Strength, durability, energy balance	Supports physical strength, promotes energy balance, hypoallergenic

Cobalt	Hormonal regulation, tissue repair, immune support	Balances hormones, supports tissue healing, enhances immune response
Stainless Steel	Hygiene, durability, general health	Prevents infections, long-lasting, hypoallergenic
Nickel	Strength, durability, resistance to corrosion	Strength, supports ligament and tendon health, promotes endurance and recovery
Palladium	Catalytic, biocompatible, antioxidant	Supports hormone regulation, reduces oxidative stress, enhances immune function

Body Systems and Corresponding Metals

Body System	Corresponding Metals	Primary Benefits
Circulatory System	Gold, Copper	Enhances blood flow, reduces inflammation, supports heart health
Respiratory System	Silver	Antimicrobial properties, reduces respiratory infections, supports lung health
Digestive System	Copper, Stainless Steel	Reduces inflammation, supports gut health, enhances nutrient absorption
Nervous System	Platinum	Enhances mental clarity, reduces stress, supports nerve function
Skeletal System	Titanium	Supports bone health, promotes tissue repair, enhances strength
Immune System	Stainless Steel	Antimicrobial properties, supports immune response, reduces inflammation
Integumentary System	Silver	Promotes skin health, reduces inflammation, supports wound healing

Reproductive System	Gold	Balances hormones, supports reproductive health, reduces inflammation
Endocrine System	Palladium	Balances hormones, supports gland function, reduces stress
Urinary System	Cobalt	Supports kidney function, reduces inflammation, prevents infections
Muscular System	Nickel	Enhances muscle strength, supports recovery, reduces inflammation
Lymphatic System	Copper, Silver	Antimicrobial properties, supports immune response, reduces inflammation

Quick Reference Chart for Body Systems and Corresponding Metals

Body System	Corresponding Metals
Circulatory System	Gold, Copper
Respiratory System	Silver
Digestive System	Copper, Stainless Steel
Nervous System	Platinum
Skeletal System	Titanium
Immune System	Stainless Steel
Integumentary System	Silver
Reproductive System	Gold
Endocrine System	Palladium
Urinary System	Cobalt
Muscular System	Nickel
Lymphatic System	Copper, Silver

Quick Reference Guide for Body Systems, Metal Rings, and Finger Placements

Based on the details from previous conversations, here is the accurate and corrected reference for body systems, their corresponding metals, and finger placements:

Circulatory System

> Metals: Gold, Copper

> Finger Placement: Ring Finger (Gold), Middle Finger (Copper)

Respiratory System

> Metals: Silver

> Finger Placement: Index Finger

Digestive System

> Metals: Copper, Stainless Steel

> Finger Placement: Middle Finger, Little Finger (Copper), Thumb, Ring Finger, Middle Finger (Stainless Steel)

Nervous System

> Metals: Platinum

> Finger Placement: Ring Finger, Middle Finger (Platinum)

Skeletal System

>Metals: Titanium

>Finger Placement: Middle Finger, Ring Finger (Titanium)

Immune System

>Metals: Stainless Steel

>Finger Placement: Little Finger, Middle Finger (Stainless Steel)

Integumentary System (Skin, Hair, Nails)

>Metals: Silver

>Finger Placement: Ring Finger, Little Finger (Silver)

Reproductive System

>Metals: Gold

>Finger Placement: Ring Finger, Index Finger (Gold

Endocrine System

>Metals: Palladium

>Finger Placement: Ring Finger, Middle Finger (Palladium)

Urinary System

> Metals: Cobalt

> Finger Placement: Middle Finger, Little Finger (Cobalt)

Muscular System

> Metals: Nickel

> Finger Placement: Thumb, Middle Finger (Nickel)

Lymphatic System

> Metals: Copper, Silver

> Finger Placement: Ring Finger, Little Finger (Copper), Ring Finger, Little Finger (Silver)

Glossary of Terms

A

Antimicrobial: Refers to substances that kill or inhibit the growth of microorganisms such as bacteria, viruses, and fungi.

Anti-inflammatory: Properties that reduce inflammation or swelling in the body.

B

Biocompatibility: The ability of a material to be compatible with living tissue without causing an immune response or rejection.

C

Catalytic Properties: The ability of a substance to accelerate a chemical reaction.

Chronic Pelvic Inflammatory Disease (PID): A long-term inflammation of the female reproductive organs caused by bacterial infection.

Conductivity: The ability of a material to conduct electricity or heat.

D

Detoxification: The process of removing toxic substances from the body.

E

Endocrine System: A collection of glands that produce hormones to regulate metabolism, growth, development, tissue function, sexual function, reproduction, sleep, and mood.

Energy Healing: A holistic practice that involves channeling healing energy to balance and heal the body, mind, and spirit.

F

Fertility Treatments: Medical treatments aimed at assisting individuals in achieving pregnancy.

H

Holistic Health: An approach to wellness that considers the whole person, including physical, emotional, mental, and spiritual aspects.

Hormonal Balance: The state of having optimal levels of hormones in the body, which are crucial for various bodily functions.

I

Immunological Memory: The ability of the immune system to remember previous encounters with pathogens and respond more effectively in future encounters.

Inflammation: The body's response to injury or infection, characterized by redness, swelling, heat, and pain.

Integumentary System: The organ system consisting of the skin, hair, nails, and associated glands.

M

Mental Clarity: The state of having a clear, focused, and unconfused mind.

Metabolism: The chemical processes that occur within a living organism to maintain life, including converting food to energy and building and repairing tissues.

N

Nanotechnology: The manipulation of matter on an atomic or molecular scale, particularly to create microscopic devices or materials.

P

Photothermal Therapy: A treatment that uses light to generate heat to target and destroy cancer cells.

Platinum: A precious metal known for its durability, biocompatibility, and ability to enhance mental clarity and emotional stability.

R

Reproductive System: The organ system responsible for producing, nurturing, and transporting reproductive cells and supporting the development of offspring.

Regenerative Medicine: A branch of medicine focused on regenerating, repairing, or replacing damaged cells, tissues, and organs.

S

Stainless Steel: An alloy known for its resistance to corrosion, durability, and use in various medical and everyday applications.

Stem Cell: A cell with the potential to develop into many different types of cells in the body, used in regenerative medicine.

T

Tissue Engineering: The use of a combination of cells, engineering, and materials methods to repair or replace biological tissues.

Traditional Chinese Medicine (TCM): An ancient system of medicine based on the balance of bodily energies and the use of herbal medicine, acupuncture, and other therapies.

W

Wound Healing: The process of repairing the skin and other tissues after injury.

V

Vitality: The state of being strong, active, and energetic, often used in reference to overall health and well-being.

Bibliography

BOOKS

Ayurveda and Metals:

- Lad, Vasant. The Complete Book of Ayurvedic Home Remedies. Harmony Books, 1999.
- Dash, Bhagwan, and Lalitesh Kashyap. Materia Medica of Ayurveda. B. Jain Publishers, 1980.

Traditional Chinese Medicine (TCM):

- Kaptchuk, Ted J. The Web That Has No Weaver: Understanding Chinese Medicine. McGraw-Hill, 2000.
- Maciocia, Giovanni. The Foundations of Chinese Medicine: A Comprehensive Text for Acupuncturists and Herbalists. Elsevier Health Sciences, 2005.

Holistic Health and Metal Therapy:

- Weil, Andrew. Spontaneous Healing: How to Discover and Enhance Your Body's Natural Ability to Maintain and Heal Itself. Knopf, 1995.
- Gerber, Richard. Vibrational Medicine: The #1 Handbook of Subtle-Energy Therapies. Bear & Company, 2001.

Metals in Modern Medicine:

- Andrews, P. C. Medicinal Inorganic Chemistry. Royal Society of Chemistry, 2010.
- Sigel, Astrid, Helmut Sigel, and Roland K. O. Sigel, eds. Metals in Biological Systems. CRC Press, 2000.

JOURNALS AND ARTICLES

Nanotechnology and Metal-Based Therapies:

- Jain, Prashant K., et al. "Gold Nanoparticles as Therapeutic Agents: Advances and Challenges." Chemical Society Reviews, vol. 41, no. 7, 2012, pp. 2849-2864.
- Murphy, Catherine J., et al. "Gold Nanoparticles in Biology: Beyond Toxicity to Cellular Imaging." Accounts of Chemical Research, vol. 41, no. 12, 2008, pp. 1721-1730.

Antimicrobial Properties of Metals:

- Lemire, Joseph A., Joe J. Harrison, and Raymond J. Turner. "Antimicrobial Activity of Metals: Mechanisms, Molecular Targets, and Applications." Nature Reviews Microbiology, vol. 11, no. 6, 2013, pp. 371-384.
- Lansdown, A. B. G. "A Review of the Use of Silver in Wound Care: Facts and Fallacies." British Journal of Nursing, vol. 13, no. 6, 2004, pp. S6-S19.

Integrative Medicine:

- Maizes, Victoria, et al. "Integrative Medicine and Patient-Centered Care." Explore: The Journal of Science and Healing, vol. 5, no. 5, 2009, pp. 277-289.
- Rakel, David, and Nancy Faass. Integrative Medicine. Saunders, 2003.

ONLINE RESOURCES
World Health Organization (WHO):

> "Traditional, Complementary and Integrative Medicine." World Health Organization, 2021. https://www.who.int/health-topics/traditional-complementary-and-integrative-medicine

National Institutes of Health (NIH):

> "Nanotechnology and Human Health." National Institute of Environmental Health Sciences, 2021. https://www.niehs.nih.gov/research/supported/exposure/nano/index.cfm

PUBMED:
- "Gold Nanoparticles for Cancer Therapy." PubMed, 2021. https://pubmed.ncbi.nlm.nih.gov/

AMERICAN HOLISTIC HEALTH ASSOCIATION (AHHA):
- "Holistic Health and Wellness Resources." AHHA, 2021. https://ahha.org/

Message from the Author,
Dr. Constance Santego

Using metal rings to balance your body systems is an incredible journey of self-discovery and healing. The techniques shared in this book are rooted in ancient wisdom and modern holistic practices, empowering you to take control of your health and well-being.

Try out the methods outlined in these pages and find the ones that resonate most with you. Trust in your ability to connect with your body's energy and make informed decisions about your health. Remember, the key lies in the questions you ask—clear, literal questions yield the most accurate responses.

Experiment with these techniques on yourself, your family, and your friends. Whether for physical health, emotional balance, or mental clarity, you'll find that these practices can enhance many aspects of your life.

Enjoy the journey!

Dr. Constance Santego

Dr. Constance Santego: A Pioneer in Holistic Health and Ring Therapy

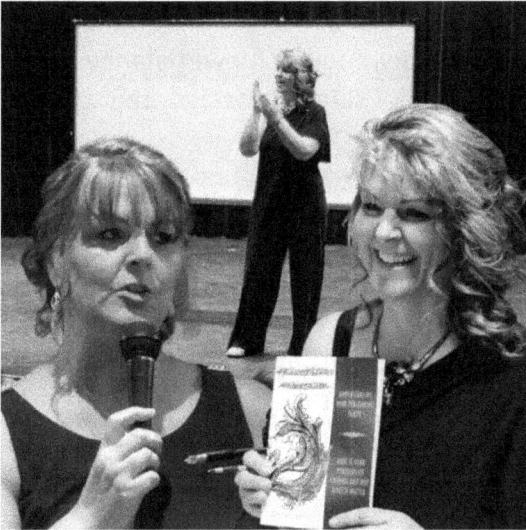

Dr. Constance Santego is a highly respected expert in the field of holistic health and spiritual healing, with over twenty-five years of experience teaching courses on these subjects. She has developed a deep understanding of the interconnectedness of the mind, body, and spirit in achieving overall well-being.

Dr. Santego holds a Ph.D. and Doctorate in Natural Medicine, which has provided her with a comprehensive understanding of alternative healing modalities and their application in promoting optimal health. Her educational background has equipped her with the knowledge to address health concerns from a holistic perspective, considering the physical, emotional, and spiritual aspects of an individual's well-being.

Throughout her career, Dr. Santego has been committed to sharing her knowledge and empowering others to take control of their health and healing. She has a unique ability to blend scientific research and traditional wisdom, creating a bridge between conventional and alternative medicine.

In addition to her expertise in various holistic practices, Dr. Santego is proficient in the field of Ring Therapy. This innovative approach combines the ancient wisdom of metals and their healing properties with modern muscle testing techniques to determine the optimal metal and finger placement for individual health concerns. Through her extensive research and practical application, Dr. Santego has developed a system that helps individuals achieve balance and well-being by wearing specific metal rings on designated fingers.

She also contributes her extensive knowledge in her "Secrets of a Healer" educational series, Dr. Santego draws upon her vast experience and expertise to captivate readers with her insights and teachings. She takes readers on a transformative journey, delving into the realms of holistic health, spirituality, and self-discovery. Through her writing, she aims to inspire individuals to tap into their own innate healing abilities and embrace a balanced and harmonious approach to well-being.

Dr. Santego's work has touched the lives of many, guiding them toward a more profound understanding of themselves and their connection to the world around them. Her series serves as a beacon of wisdom, offering practical tools and techniques for personal growth and transformation.

Overall, Dr. Constance Santego's blend of knowledge, experience, and passion makes her a captivating figure in the field of holistic health, spiritual healing, and ring therapy. Her contributions through teaching, writing, and her spellbinding series continue to inspire and empower individuals on their journeys toward well-being and self-discovery.

ALSO AVAILABLE

RING THERAPY PRACTITIONER CERTIFICATION PROGRAM

The ***Ring Therapy Practitioner Certification Program*** is a comprehensive course designed for individuals seeking to master the art of ring therapy for holistic healing. This program delves into the principles of Traditional Chinese Medicine (TCM), Ayurveda, and modern holistic practices, teaching you how to use metal rings to balance and enhance various body systems. You'll learn to apply these techniques effectively through detailed modules and hands-on practicum, providing personalized health solutions. Join us to gain valuable skills and become a certified practitioner, ready to help others achieve optimal health and well-being through ring therapy.

READ MORE:

https://constancesantego.ca/ring-therapy/

https://3jinn.com/courses/ring-therapy-practitioner-certification-program/

PLAY THE GAME *IKONA* – DISCOVER YOUR INNER GENIE

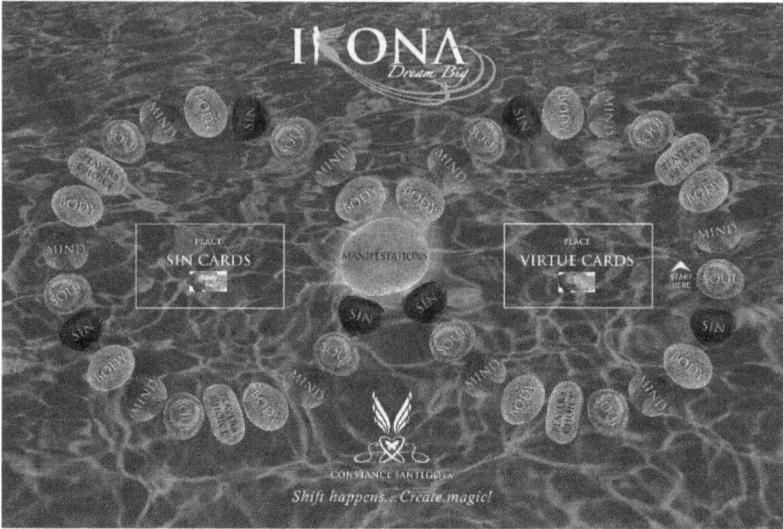

For additional information on

Constance Santego's

wide range of Motivational Products, Coaching Sessions,
Spiritual Retreats,
Live Events and Educational Programs

Go to

www.ConstanceSantego.ca

Follow on Instagram - Constance_Santego and
Facebook - constancesantegoo

Subscribe and receive Free Information and Meditations on my
YouTube Channel - Constance Santego

www.ingramcontent.com/pod-product-compliance
Lightning Source LLC
Chambersburg PA
CBHW062113020426
42335CB00013B/946